A HANDBOOK OF OBSTETRICS AND GYNAECOLOGY CARE
DURING PANDEMIC OF A NOVEL RESPIRATORY VIRUS

SOUMYA RANJAN PANDA
MBBS, MS (O & G), PDF (ENDOGYNECOLOGY)

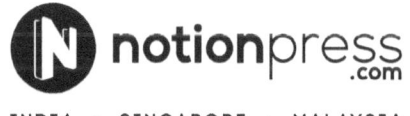

INDIA • SINGAPORE • MALAYSIA

Notion Press

No.8, 3rd Cross Street,
CIT Colony, Mylapore,
Chennai, Tamil Nadu – 600004

First Published by Notion Press 2020
Copyright © Soumya Ranjan Panda 2020
All Rights Reserved.

ISBN 978-1-63714-618-7

This book has been published with all efforts taken to make the material error-free after the consent of the author. However, the author and the publisher do not assume and hereby disclaim any liability to any party for any loss, damage, or disruption caused by errors or omissions, whether such errors or omissions result from negligence, accident, or any other cause.

While every effort has been made to avoid any mistake or omission, this publication is being sold on the condition and understanding that neither the author nor the publishers or printers would be liable in any manner to any person by reason of any mistake or omission in this publication or for any action taken or omitted to be taken or advice rendered or accepted on the basis of this work. For any defect in printing or binding the publishers will be liable only to replace the defective copy by another copy of this work then available.

Dedication

This book is dedicated to all the frontline COVID warriors who sacrifice themselves to protect our society.

Contents

Foreword   9
Preface   11
Acknowledgments   13

1. The COVID-19 pandemic   15
    1.1 Background   16
    1.2 Physicochemical Properties of SARS-COV-2   16
    1.3 Source of Infection   17
    1.4 Spectrum of Infection   17
    1.5 Conclusion   18
    1.6 References   18

2. Virology and Pathophysiology of COVID-19   21
    2.1 Coronavirus and SARS-COV-2   22
    2.2 Mechanism of SARS-CoV-2 invasion into host cells   23
    2.3 Stages of pathogenesis   24
    2.4 ACE-2 receptor expression during pregnancy   27
    2.5 References   28

3. Personal protective equipment and guidance for health care personnel.   34
    3.1 Background   35

3.2 Precautions for healthcare workers	35
3.3 Appropriate levels of PPE	37
3.4 Types of PPE masks	39
3.5 Are vaginal or cesarean deliveries aerosol-generating procedures?	43
3.6 Recommendations For Obstetric Health Care Settings To Reduce Health Care Personnel Exposure To Covid-19	44
3.7 Summary and conclusion	46
3.8 References	47
4. Susceptibility to infection and clinical manifestation	52
4.1 Effect of COVID19 on Maternal and Fetal Outcome	53
4.2 Clinical manifestations	53
4.3 Effects of COVID-19 on mother's health	55
4.4 Effects On Foetus	55
4.5 Conclusion	55
4.6 References	56
5. Place of care: Special arrangement and availability of essential facilities	58
5.1 Introduction	59
5.2 Place of care	59
5.3 Triage	60
5.4 Immediate implementation of appropriate IPC (Infection prevention and control) measures: [3]	61
5.5 Current recommendations	61
5.6 References	62

6. Antepartum, Intrapartum and Postpartum Care during COVID-19 pandemic. ... 64
   - 6.1 Introduction ... 65
   - 6.2 Diagnosis ... 65
   - 6.3 Management ... 68
   - 6.4 Management pregnant women with COVID-19 with severe/ critical illness ... 74
   - 6.5 Summary ... 77
   - 6.6 References ... 80

7. Contraceptive advice and reproductive health care during COVID-19 pandemic. ... 86
   - 7.1 Background ... 87
   - 7.2 Selected strategies for improving contraception access during the COVID-19 pandemic ... 87
   - 7.3 References ... 90

8. Laparoscopy and Hysteroscopy during COVID-19 pandemic ... 93
   - 8.1 Background ... 94
   - 8.2 General considerations ... 95
   - 8.3 Viral transmission in surgically generated smoke and aerosols ... 95
   - 8.4 Summary of current literature ... 98
   - 8.5 Recommendations for laparoscopic surgery in suspected or confirmed COVID-19 ... 99
   - 8.6 Hysteroscopy during COVID-19 pandemic: ... 104
   - 8.7 Recommendations for hysteroscopic procedures during the COVID-19 pandemic ... 105

8.8 Conclusion	107
8.9 References	108

9. Management of Gynaecological cancers during COVID-19 pandemic. — 115
   - 9.1 Background — 116
   - 9.2 General considerations — 117
   - 9.3 Cervical cancer — 118
   - 9.4 Ovarian cancer — 121
   - 9.5 Endometrial cancer — 124
   - 9.6 Gestational trophoblastic neoplasia — 126
   - 9.7 Conclusion — 126
   - 9.8 Reference — 127

10. COVID-19 pandemic and impact on Maternal psychological health — 135
    - 10.1 Background — 136
    - 10.2 The Burden of mental health during the pandemic — 137
    - 10.3 Guidance for the care of maternal psychological health.[11] — 139
    - 10.4 Conclusion — 140
    - 10.5 References — 141

Foreword

The author is a Gynecologist and Laparoscopic gynaecologic surgeon and currently working as an Assistant professor at AIIMS, Mangalagiri, Andhra Pradesh. He was quite influenced by the enthusiasm, dedicated work and sacrifices of the frontline COVID warriors during the current pandemic. In deed the COVID warriors proved again why ours is the noblest profession. This fact encouraged the author to write a book that will be helpful in tackling the current pandemic, in particular concentrating on the current recommendations of management in various aspects of Obstetrical and Gynecological care in the context of COVID-19. The author is quite hopeful that this will be very useful to the readers.

Preface

Since the first case detection of COVID-19, the disease is creating havoc not only among the general public and health care workers but also among the think tanks. A lot of unknown facts about the disease make the situation even more complicated. As far as pregnancy is concerned, due to various unclear facts about the disease process including pathophysiology, natural history, management etc the apprehension and panic for the disease still continues. Although there are a lot of articles available on the topic of COVID-19, these data are discrete and the readers find it difficult to get their requirement. In such a crisis situation our vision is to provide a detailed and complete collection of basic understandings and evidences to fulfil the gap of knowledge about practice of Obstetrics and Gynecology during the era of COVID-19. In this book, we have tried to organise the facts about COVID-19 in Obstetrics and Gynecology practice. We hope a thorough knowledge about the disease process and management protocol can be obtained after going through this book. Also it will help clinicians over the world in well tackling the pandemic.

Acknowledgments

I would like to thank a lot of people in order to providing me support to complete the writing process of the book. Thanks to Dr Jaiganesh and Dr Bitan Naik for providing me the useful input for some the contents on psychological aspects of COVID-19 of this book. Finally any kind of thanking would fall short for my parents, my wife and my little Darsh. It would not be a complete one without your costant support and encouragements.

Chapter 1
The COVID-19 pandemic

Dr. Soumya Ranjan Panda,
Assistant Professor, Department of Obstetrics and
Gynecology, AIIMS, Mangalagiri, Andhra Pradesh

Abstract

A novel coronavirus (now referred to as SARS-CoV-2) was emerged as a cause of severe respiratory illness in December of 2019 first noted in Wuhan, Hubei Province, China. A state of partial immune suppression prevails throughout pregnancy and even during period of postpartum which makes them particularly susceptible to viral infections. Till now there is a lack of literature regarding various effects of COVID 19 on pregnancy. Because this is a recently emerged viral illness, most of the knowledge about the physicochemical properties of SARS-COV-2 is derived from literatures about SARS-CoV and MERS-CoV. Currently, COVID-19 patients are found to be the main source of infection, and the severity of the disease is considered to be directly proportional to the infectivity. A critical review of the available literature, including various interim guidelines can be of particular help in understanding the disease pathophysiology and guiding the management principles.

1.1 Background

A novel coronavirus (now referred to as SARS-CoV-2) was emerged as a cause of severe respiratory illness in December of 2019 first noted in Wuhan, Hubei Province, China. The virus has been classified under betacoronavirus family closely linked to the SARS virus.[1] The first case of the COVID 19 pandemic in India was reported on 30 January 2020, originating from China. A state of partial immune suppression prevails through out pregnancy and even during period of postpartum which makes them particularly susceptible to viral infections. Till now there is a lack of literature regarding various effects of COVID 19 on pregnancy. So the clinical course and the outcome with regard to foetal and maternal health among pregnant patients infected with SARS-COV-2 is still illusive. On January 30, 2020, the World Health Organization declared the outbreak as a Public Health Emergency of International Concern and the epidemic curves are still on the rise.[3,4] As this new infection continues to spread, a lot of aprehension prevails in the society because a lot of facts are still unclear about the natural course, pathogenesis, and other effects especially on pregnant women and infants. Due to the lack of data, evidence-based guidance specific to pregnant women will take time to be developed. Based on the current information available, that pregnant women seem to have the same risk as adults who are not pregnant. As more data continue to emerge, the epidemiology and clinical course of the disease will come into sharper focus.

1.2 Physicochemical Properties of SARS-COV-2

With a diameter of around 60-100 nm the virus particle attains a round or oval shape.[5] The data on physicochemical properties of SARS-COV-2 is derived from literatures about SARS-CoV and MERS-CoV. SARS-CoV-2 can be inactivated by UV or if heated at 56 °C for 30 min. The virus is also sensitive to most disinfectants such as diethyl ether, 75% ethanol, chlorine, peracetic acid, and chloroform.[5] It has been reported that the virus is more stable on plastic and stainless steel than on copper and cardboard, and can be viable up to 72 h on these surfaces. On cardboard, the half-life of SARS-CoV-2 is longer than that of SARS-CoV and the longest viability of both viruses is on stainless steel and plastic.[6]

1.3 Source of Infection

Currently, COVID-19 patients are found to be the main source of infection, and the severity of the disease is considered to be directly proportional to the infectivity. However asymptomatic persons infected with SARS-COV-2 or patients in the incubation period are also capable of shedding the virus and also are potential sources of infection.[7]

1.4 Spectrum of Infection

Typically, COVID-19 is a type of self-limiting infectious disease. Although most cases with mild symptoms can recover in 1–2 weeks, a good proportion of patients can end up with severe disease or death especially in those having other co morbidities. COVID-19 can cause following outcomes: 1) asymptomatically infected persons (1.2%) 2) mild to medium cases (80.9%) 3) severe cases (13.8%) 4) critical case (4.7%) and 5) death (2.3%).[8] Current literature indicates that the proportion of asymptomatic infection in children under 10-years old is as high as 15.8%.[9]

The outbreak initially (8 December 2020) took place in Wuhan and its surroundings in Hubei Province. Without taking much time it crossed border and became a pandemic. Countries containing the highest cumulative confirmed cases in the world are China (24.6%), Italy (17.8%), USA (9.5%), Spain (8.6%), and Germany (7.5%). Higher case-fatality rates were found in Italy (9.3%), Iran (7.8%), and Spain (6.0%). [10]

1.5 Conclusion

At present, there is uncertainty on many aspects of the clinical course and management of COVID-19 infection in pregnancy. Hence a critical review of the available literature, including various interim guidelines can be of particular help in understanding the disease pathophysiology and guiding the management principles. In the following chapters we have discussed various queries related to COVID-19 infection in pregnancy.

1.6 References

1. Team NCPERE. Vital surveillances: the epidemiological characteristics of an outbreak of 2019 novel coronavirus diseases (COVID-19) – China. China CDC Weekly. 2020;2(8):113-22.

2. World Health Organization. Statement on the Second Meeting of the International Health Regulations. Emergency Committee regarding the outbreak of novel coronavirus (2019-nCoV); 2005. Available from: https://www.who.int/ news-room/detail/30-01-2020-statement-on-the-second meeting-of-the-

international-health-regulations-(2005)- emergency-committee-regarding-the-outbreak-of-novel coronavirus-(2019-ncov), accessed on February 17, 2020.

3. World Health Organization. Situation report-24. Geneva: WHO; 2020.

4. Lu R, Zhao X, Li J, et al. Genomic characterization and epidemiology of 2019 novel coronavirus: implications for virus origins and receptor binding. Lancet 2020; published online 30th January. https://doi.org/10.1016/S0140-6736(20)30251-8.

5. General Office of National Health Commission. General Office of National Administration of Traditional Chinese Medicine [(accessed on 20 February 2020)];Diagnostic and treatment protocol for Novel Coronavirus Pneumonia. (Trial version 6) Available online: http://www.nhc.gov.cn/yzygj/s7653p/202002/8334a8326dd94d329df351d7da8aefc2.shtml:

6. Van Doremalen N., Bushmaker T., Morris D.H., Holbrook M.G., Gamble A., Williamson B.N., Tamin A., Harcourt J.L., Thornburg N.J., Gerber S.I., et al. Aerosol and Surface Stability of SARS-CoV-2 as Compared with SARS-CoV-1. N. Engl. J. Med. 2020 doi: 10.1056/NEJMc2004973. [PMC free article] [PubMed] [CrossRef] [Google Scholar]

7. Hoehl S., Berger A., Kortenbusch M., Cinatl J., Bojkova D., Rabenau H., Behrens P., Böddinghaus B., Götsch

U., Naujoks F., et al. Evidence of SARS-CoV-2 Infection in Returning Travelers from Wuhan, China. N. Engl. J. Med. 2020 doi: 10.1056/NEJMc2001899. [PMC free article] [PubMed] [CrossRef] [Google Scholar]

8. Novel Coronavirus Pneumonia Emergency Response Epidemiology Team The epidemiological characteristics of an outbreak of 2019 novel coronavirus diseases (COVID-19) in China. Zhonghualiuxingbingxuezazhi. 2020;41:145–151. doi: 10.3760/cma.j.issn.0254-6450.2020.02.003. [PubMed] [CrossRef] [Google Scholar]

9. Lu X., Zhang L., Du H., Zhang J., Li Y.Y., Qu J., Zhang W., Wang Y., Bao S., Li Y., et al. SARS-CoV-2 Infection in Children. N. Engl. J. Med. 2020 doi: 10.1056/NEJMc2005073. [PMC free article] [PubMed] [CrossRef] [Google Scholar]

10. World Health Organization [(accessed on 23 March 2020)];Coronavirus Disease (COVID-2019) Situation Reports. Update on 24:00 of March 23. Available online: https://www.who.int/emergencies/diseases/novel-coronavirus-2019/situation-reports/

Chapter 2
Virology and Pathophysiology of COVID-19

1. Dr. Soumya Ranjan Panda,

Assistant Professor, Department of Obstetrics and Gynecology, AIIMS, Mangalagiri, Andhra Pradesh

2. Dr. Bitan Naik

Assistant Professor, Department of Pathology, IMS, BHU, Varanasi.

Abstract

Coronavirus is an enveloped, positive-sense virus with a single-stranded RNA. SARS-CoV, Middle East respiratory syndrome coronavirus (MERS-CoV) and the SARS-CoV-2 are grouped under β coronaviruses. The life cycle of the virus with the host consists of the following five steps: Attachment, Penetration, Biosynthesis, Maturation and Release. As with SARS-CoV, Angiotensin-converting enzyme 2 (ACE2) acts as a functional receptor for SARS-CoV-2 also. ACE2 expression is well documented in lung, heart, ileum, kidney and bladder. It has also been found that ACE2 is widely expressed in human placenta. COVID-19 disease confined to the conducting airways should be mild and can be treated symptomatically at home. However, COVID-19 disease that has progressed to the gas exchange units of the lung must be monitored with the utmost care.

2.1 Coronavirus and SARS-COV-2

Coronavirus is an enveloped, positive-sense virus with a single-stranded RNA and bearing a size of ~30 kb. [1] Depending upon the structure of their genome, they are largely grouped into four genera, i.e. α, β, γ, and δ. [2] The coronaviruses responsible for common cold and croup in humans, like 229E and NL63, belong to α coronavirus. On the other hand, SARS-CoV, Middle East respiratory syndrome coronavirus (MERS-CoV) and the recent sensation, SARS-CoV-2 are grouped under β coronaviruses.

Structurally coronaviruses are made up of four structural proteins (figure 2.1). These are Spike (S), membrane (M), envelop (E) and nucleocapsid (N) proteins. [3] Of these, Spike protein is the most important one as it is the protein that is responsible for the diversity of coronaviruses and host tropism. It comprises a transmembrane trimetric glycoprotein that is evident as a protrusion from the viral surface. Again, the spike protein has two functional subunits (S1 and S2). Whereas S1 subunit binds to the host cell receptor, S2 subunit is responsible for the fusion of the viral and cellular membranes.

2.2 Mechanism of SARS-CoV-2 invasion into host cells

The life cycle of the virus with the host consists of the following five steps:

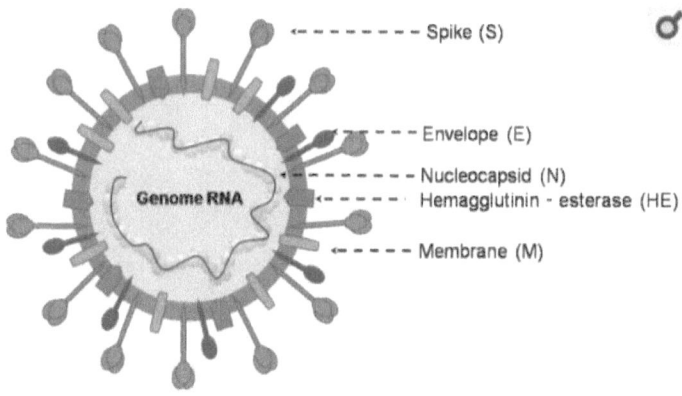

Figure-1: Beta coronavirus:[3,4] The β-coronavirus particle. β-coronavirus is an enveloped, nonsegmented, positive-sense single-stranded RNA virus with a size approximately of 29.9 kb. The virion has a nucleocapsid composed of genomic RNA, four structural proteins (Spike (S), membrane (M), envelop (E) and nucleocapsid (N) proteins) and hemagglutinin-esterase (HE).

1) Attachment: the phase of binding of viruses to host receptors,

2) Penetration: attachment is followed by a phase of penetration by gaining entrance into the host cells through endocytosis or membrane fusion.

3) Biosynthesis: Once viral contents are released inside the host cells, viral RNA enters the nucleus for replication. Viral mRNA is used to biosynthesize viral proteins.

4) Maturation: Then, new viral particles are produced and

5) Release.

As with SARS-CoV, Angiotensin-converting enzyme 2 (ACE2) acts as a functional receptor for SARS-CoV-2 also.[5-8] ACE2 expression is well documented in lung, heart, ileum, kidney and bladder. [9] Additional targets for SARS-CoV-2 are still unknown and needs further investigation. After the binding of SARS-CoV-2 to the host protein, a cleavage by protease ensues involving the spike protein to activate it. To describe this action, a two-step sequential protease cleavage to activate spike protein of SARS-CoV and MERS-CoV was proposed as a model. This consists of cleavage at the S1/S2 cleavage site and cleavage for activation at the S'2 site, a position adjacent to a fusion peptide within the S2 subunit.[10-12] Subsequent to the second cleavage at the S'2 site, presumably there is the activation of the spike for membrane fusion via irreversible, conformational changes. The coronavirus spike is unusual among viruses because a range of different proteases can cleave and activate it. [13] The presence of furin cleavage site ("RPPA" sequence) at the S1/S2 site is a unique characteristic of SARS-CoV-2 compared to other coronaviruses. the S1/S2 site was also subjected to cleavage by other proteases such as transmembrane protease serine 2 (TMPRSS2) and cathepsin L.[12,14] However, the ubiquitous expression of furin likely makes this virus extremely pathogenic.

2.3 Stages of pathogenesis

Pathogenesis of COVID-19 can be grossly divided into three phases based upon the cells that are likely infected. [15]

Stage 1: Stage of Asymptomatic state (initial 1–2 days of infection):

After binding to epithelial cells in the nasal cavity, the inhaled virus starts replicating. ACE2 is the primary receptor for both SARS-CoV2 and SARS-CoV.[14,16] Although there is local propagation of the virus, there is the development of a limited innate immune response. At this stage, we can detect the virus by nasal swabs. Albeit a low viral burden, these individuals are infectious. One can find the RT-PCR value for the viral RNA to be of useful value to predict the viral load, the subsequent infectivity and clinical course.

Stage 2: stage of Upper airway and conducting airway response (next few days)

Gradually, the virus propagates and migrates down the respiratory tract along the conducting airways. At this stage, a more robust innate immune response is triggered. The virus can be detected through nasal swabs or sputum. At the same time, early markers of the innate immune response can also be helpful in diagnosis. During this time, the clinical manifestations of COVID-19 are evident. The level of CXCL10, an innate response cytokine may be predictive of the subsequent clinical course.[17] It has been found that epithelial cells those are Virally infected, are a major source of beta and lambda interferons.[18] CXCL10 is thought to be an interferon responsive gene.[19,20]The subsequent course of the disease can be predicted by measuring the level of the host innate immune response. About 80% of the patients infected with SARS- COV-2 will experience a mild disease, mostly limited to the upper and conducting airways.[15]

Stage 3: stage of Hypoxia, ground-glass infiltrates, and progression to ARDS:

This is really unfortunate that nearly 20% of the infected patients may progress to stage 3 disease acquiring development of pulmonary infiltrates. A portion of these may end up in developing very severe disease. After reaching the gas exchange units of the lung, the virus preferentially infects alveolar type II cells compared to type-I cells. This preference of alveolar cell types is in line with both SARS-CoV and influenza.[21,22] Generally, the infected alveolar units are peripheral and subpleural.[23,24] a Large number of viral particles are released subsequent to virus multiplication. Ultimately, there is apoptosis of the infected cells.[19] Maintaining the same path the released viral particles can infect type II cells in adjacent units and the worsening of lung tissue damage continues. In response to the above process, the secondary pathway for epithelial regeneration will be triggered. This sequence of events has been postulated based on the murine model of influenza pneumonia.[25,26] A diffuse alveolar damage associated with fibrin rich hyaline membranes and a few multinucleated giant cells are the pathological end result of SARS and COVID-19 infection. [27,28] More severe scarring and fibrosis may result than other forms of ARDS. This is due to the process leading to an aberrant wound healing. Recovery requires the development of a vigorous innate and acquired immune response leading to epithelial regeneration. Owing to their diminished immune response reduced ability to repair the damaged epithelium and reduced mucociliary clearance, the elderly individuals are particularly at increased risk of severe infection.[29]

This pathogenesis model is mostly based on the assumption that viral entry by SARS-CoV-2 will be the same as SARS-CoV. Till the time, detailed studies on infection and the innate immune response of differentiated primary human lung cells are available the above-highlighted points can help us in understanding the disease process.

2.4 ACE-2 receptor expression during pregnancy

It has been found that ACE2 is widely expressed in human placenta.[30] In placental villi, ACE2 is expressed in various levels of cells like syncytiotrophoblast, cytotrophoblast, endothelium and vascular smooth muscle of primary and secondary villi. It's also found in various parts of the maternal stroma like invading and intravascular trophoblast and in decidual cells as well as in arterial and venous endothelium and smooth muscle of the umbilical cord.[30] Furthermore, *ACE2* reaches the highest level in early gestation.[31] As per the GeneCards, ACE2 expression in the placenta is even greater than that found in the lung, suggesting a good possibility of viral infection of the placenta. There are instances where early-onset SARS-VOV-2 infection was identified in infants whose nasopharyngeal and anal swabs were found to be positive on Day 2 and 4 of life.[32] In another report, a neonate born to a mother with COVID-19 infection was found to have elevated IgM antibodies at two h after birth.[33] Given that the identification of 2019-nCoV in human airway epithelial cells requires at least 96 h of culture (National Health Commission of the People's Republic of China, 2020), we speculate that intrauterine infection with SARS-COV-2 may appear and the foetuses may be infected during gestation. However, there is no direct evidence of vertical transmission till now, and also there is no evidence of foetal affection.

In conclusion, COVID-19 disease confined to the conducting airways should be mild and can be treated symptomatically at home. However, COVID-19 disease that has progressed to the gas exchange units of the lung must be monitored with the utmost care and supported to the best of our ability, as we await the development and testing of specific antiviral drugs.

2.5 References

1. Channappanavar R, Zhao J, Perlman S. T cell-mediated immune response to respiratory coronaviruses. Immunol Res. 2014 Aug;59(1-3):118-28. doi: 10.1007/s12026-014-8534-z. PMID: 24845462; PMCID: PMC4125530.

2. Rabi FA, Al Zoubi MS, Kasasbeh GA, Salameh DM, Al-Nasser AD. SARS-CoV-2 and Coronavirus Disease 2019: What We Know So Far. Pathogens. 2020 Mar 20;9(3):231. doi: 10.3390/pathogens9030231. PMID: 32245083; PMCID: PMC7157541.

3. Bosch BJ, van der Zee R, de Haan CA, Rottier PJ. The coronavirus spike protein is a class I virus fusion protein: structural and functional characterization of the fusion core complex. J Virol. 2003 Aug;77(16):8801-11. doi: 10.1128/jvi.77.16.8801-11.2003. PMID: 12885899; PMCID: PMC167208.

4. 4.Weiss S.R., Leibowitz J.L. Coronavirus pathogenesis. Adv. Virus Res. 2011;81:85–164. doi: 10.1016/b978-0-12-385885-6.00009-2. [PMC free article] [PubMed] [CrossRef] [Google Scholar]

5. Li W, Moore MJ, Vasilieva N, Sui J, Wong SK, Berne MA et al., Angiotensin-converting enzyme 2 is a functional receptor for the SARS coronavirus. Nature. 2003 Nov 27;426(6965):450-4. doi: 10.1038/nature02145. PMID: 14647384; PMCID: PMC7095016.

6. Chen Y, Guo Y, Pan Y, Zhao ZJ. Structure analysis of the receptor binding of 2019-nCoV. Biochem Biophys Res Commun. 2020 Feb 17;525(1):135–40. doi: 10.1016/j.bbrc.2020.02.071. Epub ahead of print. PMID: 32081428; PMCID: PMC7092824.

7. Walls AC, Park YJ, Tortorici MA, Wall A, McGuire AT, Veesler D. Structure, Function, and Antigenicity of the SARS-CoV-2 Spike Glycoprotein. Cell. 2020 Apr 16;181(2):281-292.e6. doi: 10.1016/j.cell.2020.02.058. Epub 2020 Mar 9. PMID: 32155444; PMCID: PMC7102599.

8. Letko M, Marzi A, Munster V. Functional assessment of cell entry and receptor usage for SARS-CoV-2 and other lineage B betacoronaviruses. Nat Microbiol. 2020 Apr;5(4):562-569. doi: 10.1038/s41564-020-0688-y. Epub 2020 Feb 24. PMID: 32094589; PMCID: PMC7095430.

9. Zou X, Chen K, Zou J, Han P, Hao J, Han Z. Single-cell RNA-seq data analysis on the receptor ACE2 expression reveals the potential risk of different human organs vulnerable to 2019-nCoV infection. Front Med. 2020 Apr;14(2):185-192. doi: 10.1007/s11684-020-0754-0. Epub 2020 Mar 12. PMID: 32170560; PMCID: PMC7088738.

10. Belouzard S, Chu VC, Whittaker GR. Activation of the SARS coronavirus spike protein via sequential proteolytic cleavage at two distinct sites. Proc Natl Acad Sci U S A. 2009 Apr 7;106(14):5871-6. doi: 10.1073/pnas.0809524106. Epub 2009 Mar 24. PMID: 19321428; PMCID: PMC2660061.

11. Millet JK, Whittaker GR. Host cell entry of Middle East respiratory syndrome coronavirus after two-step, furin-mediated activation of the spike protein. Proc Natl Acad Sci U S A. 2014 Oct 21;111(42):15214-9. doi: 10.1073/pnas.1407087111. Epub 2014 Oct 6. PMID: 25288733; PMCID: PMC4210292.

12. Ou X, Liu Y, Lei X, Li P, Mi D, Ren L, Guo L, Guo R, Chen T, Hu J, Xiang Z, Mu Z, Chen X, Chen J, Hu K, Jin Q, Wang J, Qian Z. Characterization of spike glycoprotein of SARS-CoV-2 on virus entry and its immune cross-reactivity with SARS-CoV. Nat Commun. 2020 Mar 27;11(1):1620. doi: 10.1038/s41467-020-15562-9. PMID: 32221306; PMCID: PMC7100515.

13. Belouzard S, Millet JK, Licitra BN, Whittaker GR. Mechanisms of coronavirus cell entry mediated by the viral spike protein. Viruses. 2012 Jun;4(6):1011-33. doi: 10.3390/v4061011. Epub 2012 Jun 20. PMID: 22816037; PMCID: PMC3397359.

14. Hoffmann M, Kleine-Weber H, Schroeder S, et al. SARS-CoV-2 cell entry depends on ACE2 and TMPRSS2 and is blocked by a clinically proven protease inhibitor. Cell 2020; in press https://doi.org/10.1016/j.cell.2020.02.052.

15. Wu Z, McGoogan JM. Characteristics of and important lessons from the coronavirus disease 2019 (COVID-19) outbreak in China: summary of a report of 72314 cases from the Chinese Center for Disease Control and Prevention. JAMA 2020; in press.

16. Wan Y, Shang J, Graham R, et al. Receptor recognition by novel coronavirus from Wuhan: An analysis based on decade-long structural studies of SARS. J Virol 2020; 94: e00127-20.

17. Tang NL, Chan PK, Wong CK, et al. Early enhanced expression of interferon-inducible protein-10 (CXCL-10) and other chemokines predicts adverse outcome in severe acute respiratory syndrome. Clin Chem 2005; 51: 2333–2340.

18. Hancock AS, Stairiker CJ, Boesteanu AC, et al. Transcriptome analysis of infected and bystander type 2 alveolar epithelial cells during influenza A virus infection reveals in vivo Wnt pathway downregulation. J Virol 2018; 92: e01325-18.

19. Qian Z, Travanty EA, Oko L, et al. Innate immune response of human alveolar type II cells infected with severe acute respiratory syndrome-coronavirus. Am J Respir Cell Mol Biol 2013; 48: 742–748.

20. Wang J, Nikrad MP, Phang T, et al. Innate immune response to influenza A virus in differentiated human alveolar type II cells. Am J Respir Cell Mol Biol 2011; 45: 582–591.

21. Mossel EC, Wang J, Jeffers S, et al. SARS-CoV replicates in primary human alveolar type II cell cultures but not in type I-like cells. Virology 2008; 372: 127–135.

22. Weinheimer VK, Becher A, Tonnies M, et al. Influenza A viruses target type II pneumocytes in the human lung. J Infect Dis 2012; 206: 1685–1694.

23. Wu J, Wu X, Zeng W, et al. Chest CT findings in patients with corona virus disease 2019 and its relationship with clinical features. Invest Radiol 2020; in press.

24. Zhang S, Li H, Huang S, et al. High-resolution CT features of 17 cases of corona virus disease 2019 in Sichuan province, China. Eur Respir J 2020; in press.

25. Kumar PA, Hu Y, Yamamoto Y, et al. Distal airway stem cells yield alveoli in vitro and during lung regeneration following H1N1 influenza infection. Cell 2011; 147: 525–538.

26. Yee M, Domm W, Gelein R, et al. Alternative progenitor lineages regenerate the adult lung depleted of alveolar epithelial type 2 cells. Am J Respir Cell Mol Biol 2017; 56: 453–464.

27. Gu J, Korteweg C. Pathology and pathogenesis of severe acute respiratory syndrome. Am J Pathol 2007; 170: 1136–1147.

28. Xu Z, Shi L, Wang Y, et al. Pathological findings of COVID-19 associated with acute respiratory distress syndrome. Lancet Respir Med 2020; 8: 420–422.

29. Ho JC, Chan KN, Hu WH, et al. The effect of aging on nasal mucociliary clearance, beat frequency, and

ultrastructure of respiratory cilia. Am J Respir Crit Care Med 2001; 163: 983–988.

30. Valdes G , Neves LA , Anton L , Corthorn J , Chacon C , Germain AM , Merrill DC , Ferrario CM , Sarao R , Penninger J et al. Distribution of angiotensin-(1-7) and ACE2 in human placentas of normal and pathological pregnancies. *Placenta*.2006;27:200–7

31. Pringle KG, Tadros MA, Callister RJ, Lumbers ER. The expression and localization of the human placental prorenin/renin-angiotensin system throughout pregnancy: roles in trophoblast invasion and angiogenesis? Placenta. 2011 Dec;32(12):956-62. doi: 10.1016/j.placenta.2011.09.020. Epub 2011 Oct 20. PMID: 22018415.

32. Zeng L, Xia S, Yuan W, et al. Neonatal Early-Onset Infection With SARS-CoV-2 in 33 Neonates Born to Mothers With COVID-19 in Wuhan, China. *JAMA Pediatr.* 2020;174(7):722–725. doi:10.1001/jamapediatrics.2020.0878

33. Dong L, Tian J, He S, et al. Possible Vertical Transmission of SARS-CoV-2 From an Infected Mother to Her Newborn. *JAMA*. 2020;323(18):1846–1848. doi:10.1001/jama.2020.4621.

Chapter 3
Personal protective equipment and guidance for health care personnel.

Dr. Soumya Ranjan Panda,

Assistant Professor, Department of Obstetrics and Gynecology, AIIMS, Mangalagiri, Andhra Pradesh

Abstract

Obstetricians have a limited option for postponing surgery. This owes to the fact that most surgeries those are dealt with by the obstetricians are related to childbirth or some obstetrical emergencies. Airborne precaution should be used while getting involved in an aerosol-generating procedure. There are three types of precautions, i.e. contact, droplet and airborne precautions. Healthcare workers are regarded as the backbone of any healthcare system. The ongoing COVID-19 pandemic has the potential to inflict major damage to the health care system by infecting substantial health care personnel. Healthcare workers should follow the three principles to prevent acquiring the infection. These are distancing, use of appropriate PPE correctly and chemoprophylaxis. The scrupulous hand-washing facility, decontamination strategies, triage facility should be readily available in health care settings.

3.1 Background

Amid the ongoing pandemic, when most of the clinical organisations are in the discussion of postponing all elective surgeries, obstetricians have a limited option for postponing surgery. This owes to the fact that most surgeries those are dealt with by the obstetricians are related to childbirth or some obstetrical emergencies. Thus, they are the ones who are more prone to be placed in the frontline in the fight against COVID-19. Hence it's very important in part of an obstetrician to be well versed with the norms and standards to minimise the risk of contracting COVID-19 while providing their invaluable service. Of course, we have to face certain challenges in terms of shortages in supplies of personal protective equipment. Moreover, since the beginning of this pandemic, health care personnel appear to be more confusing and anxious because of the lack of knowledge on the transmission and evolution of this disease. This chapter is aimed at reviewing our current knowledge on personal protective equipment in the context of transmission of COVID-19.

3.2 Precautions for healthcare workers

Healthcare workers are regarded as the backbone of any healthcare system. The ongoing COVID-19 pandemic has the potential to inflict major damage to the health care system by infecting substantial health care personnel. Thus, particularly healthcare workers are highly vulnerable to acquire the COVID-19 infection. This is due to the fact that they have to come in contact with large numbers of patients, close contact and procedures involving spray/aerosolisation (labour, delivery, surgical procedures). In turn, the infection can spread in the other direction, i.e. from health care workers to the general population. Hence to adopt appropriate precaution while dealing with suspected or confirmed COVID-19 patients should be the norm for health care workers during this pandemic. In Italy, about 20% of healthcare workers are infected who cared for COVID-19 infected patients. [1] However, there are some positive data from Singapore and Hong Kong that with adequate use of Personal protective equipment (PPE) and other forms of infection control measures, the rate of transmission to healthcare workers is almost nil.[2]

Healthcare workers should follow the three principles to prevent acquiring the infection. These are distancing, use of appropriate PPE correctly and chemoprophylaxis. Social distancing is one of the cornerstones of prevention can't be overemphasised and should be adopted by healthcare workers whenever possible. The following measures may be helpful in this regard.

- To maintain a distance of at least 1 meter from patients and other healthcare workers. However, this may not be feasible in certain situations like clinical examination or procedures.

- To decrease the risk of fomite related spread, the consulting or examination room should be free from non-essential items.

- The practice of regular hand cleaning with soap and water or alcohol-based rubs for at least 20 seconds should be adopted.

- Patients should be offered surgical masks if they have respiratory symptoms.

In addition to the standard precautions, some enhanced precautions in the form of personal protective equipment are also essential to contain the spread of infection while caring for the suspected or confirmed COVID-19 patients presenting in labour or for those who need procedures like surgery. The PPE should include masks such as the N95 respirator (of appropriate size) and face protection by a face shield or at least goggles and other measures.[3]

3.3 Appropriate levels of PPE

At present, there is a use of multiple terms to describe PPE, which appears inconsistent and may lead to confusion. A nomenclature that describes the level of protection according to the mode of transmission should help to combat these issues and will give clarity. One such type of classification as described by Cook et al. is summarised in Table 1.[4]

According to this nomenclature, there are three types of precautions, i.e. contact, droplet and airborne precautions. Contact precaution is recommended for staffs working in the same room with designated for COVID-19 patients, and where no form of aerosol-generating procedures are undertaken, but who remain more than two metres from the patient. It's appropriate to use Droplet precaution while caring for a patient in close contact or within two metres of distance. Depending on the risk assessment, an eyewear can be added. A fluid-resistant surgical facemask is also advised for the patient. Airborne precaution should be used while getting involved in an aerosol-generating procedure. Eye protection may be via the use of goggles or a visor. Personal spectacles are insufficient.

The above-described levels of protection are incremental, i.e. droplet precautions can also prevent contact transmission. Similarly airborne precautions can also prevent droplet and contact transmission. Public Health England advises airborne precautions should be used in 'hot spots' where aerosol-generating procedures are regularly performed, for any suspected COVID19 patients. These include places of care such as intensive care unit, operating theatres where aerosol-generating procedures are done, and emergency department resuscitation areas.[5]

TABLE NO.1

Types of PPE precautions according to the mode of transmission as reported by Cook et al.[4]

Type of precaution according to the mode of transmission	Setting	Components of PPE
Contact precautions	> 2 m away from the patient	Gloves Apron
Droplet precautions	Within 2 m of patient	Gloves Apron Fluid-resistant surgical mask Eye protection (risk assess)
Airborne precautions	Aerosol generating procedure	Gloves Fluid-repellent long sleeved gown Eye protection FFP3 mask

Many organisations including the World Health Organization[6], the European Centre for Disease Control [7], Public Health England[5] and the European Society of Intensive Care Medicine and Society of Critical Care Medicine[8] have produced guidance on PPE which are grossly consistent. According to these guidelines, airborne precautions comprises fit-tested and fit-checked high filtration mask, goggles or visor, long-sleeved fluid repellent gown and gloves. Though few of the current guidelines state in favour of using FFP3 masks,[5] most of these guidelines recommend to use of FFP2 masks.[6,7,9]

3.4 Types of PPE masks

Nomenclature of masks and respirators is essential to understand as various classifications are used by different standards, and without this knowledge one may land up in unwanted confusion. Here is a brief summary describing the nomenclature and types of masks and respirators.

Face masks

The face mask is a loose-fitting disposable mask that creates a physical barrier between the wearer's nose and mouth and contaminants. Also known as medical or surgical masks and are classified into Type I, Type II or Type IIR.

Classification of Type I and Type II masks, is according to their Bacterial Filtration Efficiency (BFE). The BFE is directly related to the amount of bacteria released through the mask and into the environment. Again, depending upon the splash or fluid resistance pressure, the Type II masks are further classified into Type-II or Type-II R. Here the letter 'R' denotes splash resistance which determines the mask's resistance level to potentially contaminated fluid splashes. Hence while a type IIR mask is a splash-resistant variety, the type II mask is devoid of this property.

So, a splash or fluid-resistant (Type-IIR) surgical facemask is used to protect against droplets. It minimises dispersal of large respiratory droplets and protects against both droplet and contact transmission.[10] It's estimated to reduce the risk of transmission by at least 80%. [5]

Respirators

A respiratory protective device designed to achieve a very close facial fit and very efficient filtration of airborne particles. Also known as Filtering Face Piece.

The terms filtering facepiece FFP2, FFP3 and N95 are used to refer high performance filtering masks. The filtration is achieved via a combination of a web of polypropylene microfibres and electrostatic charge.

Grossly Filtering Face Piece respirators are classified differently by American and European standards. Going by the American standard, managed by "The US National Institute for Occupational Safety and Health (NIOSH)" which is a part of the Center for Disease Control (CDC), filtering facepiece respirators (FFRs) are classified into nine categories (N95, N99, N100, P95, P99, P100, R95, R99, and R100). The classification into 'N', 'R' and 'P' depends on their property of oil resistance. Here the letters 'N', 'R' and 'P' represent not resistant to oil, somewhat resistant to oil and strongly resistant to oil respectively. Thus the 'N' respirators cannot be used in an oil droplet environment while the 'P' respirators are best suited for oil environment. The designations in numerical such as 95, 99, and 100 show the filter's minimum filtration efficiency (the minimal percentage of particles that can be filtered under test conditions) with 95%, 99%, and 99.97%, respectively.[11]

On the other hand, Europe uses two different standards. While the EN 143 standard covers P1/P2/P3 ratings, the European standard EN 149 + A1:2009, includes three levels of protection, i.e. FFP1, FFP2 and FFP3.[12] Both standards are maintained by CEN (European Committee for Standardization). This classification is based on the individual protection factor of the type of mask, which indicates the degree to which the mask will filter out the quantity of the hazardous substances. For FFP1, FFP2 and FFP3, these factors are 4-, 10- and 20-fold, respectively.[13] Various other properties of these respirators are described in table no.2. To check the efficiency, these tests are performed on masks as delivered and during simulated use. The overall filter efficiency described for FFP1, FFP2 and FFP3 masks is 80%, 94% and 99% respectively.[12] Fluid resistance should be an essential quality of these masks if used for medical purposes. For effective use, the FFP2/3 and N95 masks should fit well to the face and create a seal. Therefore, it's important to direct individual mask fit-testing by all relevant members of staff before they are worn on clinical duty. If done properly, mask fit-testing should have a failure rate of < 5%. Any amount of higher failure rate should bring into question whether the correct testing procedure is being undertaken. As testing of these respirators is done under worse conditions of high airflow and using high penetrating aerosols (0.3-micrometre diameter), the actual Filtration performance during day to day use is likely to be higher than indicated. According to the WHO, the undamaged FFP2/3 and N95 masks can provide protection for up to 4 h, which is the approximate median tolerance time for healthcare workers. [14, 15]

TABLE NO. 2
Types of PPE masks

European standard (EN 149:2001)	European standard (EN 143) equivalent	American standard (NIOSH) equivalent	The total inward leak of particles	Protection factor (the degree to which the mask will reduce the concentration of the hazardous substance)	Mean inward leak in 8 of 10 wearers	Penetration of test aerosols (both saline and paraffin oils)	overall filter efficiency
FFP1	P1		25 %	Fourfold	22 %	20 %	80%
FFP2	P2		11 %	Tenfold	8 %	6 %	94%
		N-95					95%
FFP3		N-99	5 %	20 fold	2 %	1 %	99%
	P3						99.95%
		N-100					99.97%

3.5 Are vaginal or cesarean deliveries aerosol-generating procedures?

Recently a lot of discussion and debate is being encountered about which obstetrics procedures constitute an aerosolising procedure. Because N95 masks are advocated to be worn when aerosol-generating procedures are performed,[16], it is important to be able to identify procedures capable of producing aerosols. Intubation for general anaesthesia has been shown to produce aerosols and may increase the risk of transmission to the person performing the intubation. By contrast, cesarean deliveries under neuraxial anaesthesia (i.e., spinal or epidural) are unlikely to produce aerosols. Of late, there has been speculation on the ability to generate aerosol during the labored breathing and expulsive efforts of pushing in the second stage of labour. As we know, most of the procedures capable of generating aerosols (e.g., intubation, bronchoscopy) involve direct manipulation of the respiratory tract.[17, 18] However, of the role of turbulent gas clouds in COVID-19 transmission (as in laboured breathing) is not known.[19] Moreover, there is a paucity of data for the risks of aerosolisation during vaginal delivery. Given the limitations of the current evidence, it is not possible to definitely state whether or not aerosols are generated during the second stage of labour. However, there is no confusion on the fact that transmission of COVID-19 can occur through respiratory droplets. Hence all women with COVID-19 infection should be advised to wear a facemask during their entire hospitalisation, including during the second stage of labour (source control) whenever possible.

3.6 Recommendations For Obstetric Health Care Settings To Reduce Health Care Personnel Exposure To Covid-19

Although personal protective equipment is a vital strategy to protect health care workers, it's not the sole one, and implementation of other strategies is crucial for maximum protection. **Case finding** is one such strategy and is critical to prevent exposure in health care settings. Ideally, before entering an ambulatory care setting, pregnant patients need to be screened telephonically for possible symptoms of COVID-19 or exposures to patients with known or suspected COVID-19. [20] If an outpatient appointment is deemed essential, a facemask should be placed on any patient with respiratory symptoms immediately on presentation (known as source control), and she should be quickly isolated.

Triage areas should be separate, well-ventilated areas, and should have barriers ensuring that patients are separated (eg, plexiglass barriers) from staff during the screening process. At least six feet of physical distance should be maintained between patients in triage areas. Triage areas, waiting rooms, and patient care areas should be provided with ample of hand hygiene dispensers.

Hand hygiene is a key and crucial step for preventing nosocomial transmission of COVID-19, especially with the demonstration that virus can survive on surfaces from several hours up to 3 days depending on the surface material.[21] Furthermore, frequent cleaning of surfaces and rooms should be undertaken, with high-touch areas such as door knobs, faucets, and chair arms being wiped with an appropriate disinfectant between patients.

The number of visitors and caring personnel of a patient with suspected or confirmed COVID-19 infection should be minimised.

Use of appropriate personal protective equipment is a fundamental strategy for the protection of health care workers. as suggested by the Centers for Disease Control and Prevention (CDC) it is prudent to include an N95 respirator if available (or facemask if not available), eye protection, gown, and gloves as PPE for the care of persons with known or suspected COVID-19 infection.[16,22] For settings in which airborne transmission is the primary transmission mechanism, there are three respirator options. An N95 respirator should filter out at least 95% of airborne particles sized 0.3 micrometres in diameter, although, in practice, up to 10% of N95 respirator users exposed to aerosolised influenza had breakthrough leakage.20 Another type of respirator is a powered air-purifying respirator, which uses high-efficiency particulate air filters. These respirators are reusable and must be cleaned and disinfected after each use. Filters should be replaced according to the manufacturer's recommendations. However, the National Institute for Occupational Safety and Health has cautioned against the use of powered air-purifying respirators in the operating room because of concerns that unfiltered exhaled air may contaminate the sterile field and the absence of scientific evidence to support use. Cartridge air-purifying respirators are another option. Depending on the filter cartridge chosen, they can provide a similar level of respiratory protection to that provided by an N95 respirator and can be reused. However, communication with patients may be difficult during use, and there are no manufacturer instructions for decontamination. A facemask is a standard FDA-cleared medical mask that may or may not have a plastic face shield attached; these are the standard masks used on labour and delivery units. Surgical masks prevent transmission of viruses transmitted by large droplets, a common method for prevention of transmission of viral respiratory illnesses. [23] Importantly, whether a medical mask or respirator, the operator must wear facial protection correctly and use eye protection to assure that all mucous membranes are covered.

3.7 Summary and conclusion:

The following points can be summarised for the prevention of cross-infection.

1) PPE should not be considered as an absolute infection control measure as it is only one part of a system to prevent contamination for those working near patients with COVID-19 which might then pose a risk to those staff, other staff and patients. Other elements of a system to reduce cross-infection include

2) Avoidance of patients, visitors or staff who have or have been exposed to COVID-19 entering hospitals without reason.

3) Scrupulous hand-washing and personal hygiene.

4) Managing patients with known or suspected COVID-19 entirely separately from those without it, through isolation or cohorting.

5) Restricting personnel (both staff and visitors) in the location of patients with COVID-19 to only those who are needed.

6) Cleaning regimens with least twice daily decontamination of surfaces and equipment.

7) Minimising unnecessary patient and surface contact during patient care.

8) Best practice in donning, doffing and disposal of PPE.

9) Appropriate disposal of all single-use equipment after use and decontamination of reusable equipment strictly in line with the manufacturer's instructions.

10) Appropriate waste management.

3.8 References

1) COVID-19: Protecting Health-Care Workers. Editorial. 10228, : The Lancet, 2020, Vol. 395. https://doi.org/10.1016/S0140-6736(20)30644-9 .

2. Gawande, Atul. Keeping the Coronavirus from Infection Health-Care Workers. [Newspaper Webpage] New York : The New Yorker, 2020. https://www.newyorker.com/news/news-desk/keeping-the-coronavirus-frominfecting-health-care-workers.

3. Center for Disease Control, USA. [Online] [Cited: March 28, 2020.] https://www.newyorker.com/news/news-desk/keeping-the-coronavirus-from-infecting-health-care-workers.

4. Cook T. Personal protective equipment during the coronavirus disease (COVID) 2019 pandemic – a narrative review. Anaesthesia. 2020;75(7):920-927.

5. Public Health England. COVID-19: infection prevention and control guidance. 2020. https://www.gov.uk/government/pub lications/wuhan-novel-coronavirus-infection-prevention-and-co ntrol/wuhan-novel-coronavirus-wn-cov-infection-preventionand-control-guidance#mobile-healthcare-equipment (accessed 25/03/2020).

6. World Health Organization. Clinical management of severe acute respiratory infection when novel coronavirus (nCoV) infection is suspected. 2020. https://www.who.int/publicationsdetail/clinical-management-of-severe-acute-respiratory-infec tion-when-novel-coronavirus-(ncov)-infection-is-suspected (accessed 26/03/2020).

7. European Centre for Disease Prevention and Control. Infection prevention and control for COVID-19 in healthcare settings. 2020. https://www.ecdc.europa.eu/en/publications-data/infec tion-prevention-and-control-covid-19-healthcare-settings (accessed 31/03/2020).

8. Public Health England. When to use a surgical face mask or FFP3 respirator. 2020. https://assets.publishing.service.gov.uk/government/uploads/system/uploads/attachment_data/file /874411/When_to_use_face_mask_or_FFP3.pdf (accessed 26/ 03/2020).

9. Alhazzani W, Hylander Møller M, Arabi YM, et al. Surviving Sepsis Campaign: guidelines on the

management of critically ill adults with coronavirus disease 2019 (COVID-19). Intensive Care Medicine 2020. Epub ahead of print 28 March. https://doi.org/10.1007/s00134-020-06022-5.

10. Leung NHL, Chu DKW, Shiu EYC, et al. Respiratory virus shedding in exhaled breath and efficacy of face masks. Nature Medicine 2020. Epub 3 April. https://doi.org/10.1038/s41591- 020-0843-2 (accessed 08/04/2020).

11. NIOSH Guide to the Selection and Use of Particulate Respirators. Centres for disease control and prevention. DHHS (NIOSH) Publication Number 96-101. 1996. https://www.cdc.gov/ niosh/docs/96-101/default.html (accessed 26/03/2020).

12. BS EN 149:2001+A1:2009 Respiratory Protective Devices. Filtering half masks to protect against particles. Requirements, testing, marking. British Standard Institute. 2009. https:// www.bsigroup.com/en-GB/topics/novel-coronavirus-covid19/medical-devices-ppe/ (accessed 28/03/2020).

13. Gawn J, Clayton M, Makison C, Crook B Evaluating the protection afforded by surgical masks against influenza bioaerosols Gross protection of surgical masks compared to filtering facepiece respirators Prepared by the Health and Safety Laboratory for the Health and Safety Executive HSE Books. 2008. https://www.hse.gov.uk/research/rrpdf/rr619.pdf (accessed 26/03/2020).

14. World Health organisation. Rational use of personal protective equipment (PPE) for coronavirus disease

(COVID-19). 2020. https://apps.who.int/iris/bitstream/handle/10665/331498/ WHO-2019-nCoV-IPCPPE_use-2020.2-eng.pdf?sequence=1&isAllowed=y (accessed 26/03/2020).

15. Radonovich LJ Jr, Cheng J, Shenal BV, Hodgson M, Bender BS. Respirator tolerance in health care workers. Journal of the American Medical Association 2009; 301: 36–8. 16.17. Centers for Disease Control and Prevention. Interim infection prevention and control recommendations for patients with suspected or confirmed coronavirus disease 2019 (COVID-19) in healthcare settings. Available at: https://www.cdc.gov/coronavirus/2019-ncov/hcp/infection-control-recommendations.html. Retrieved April 1, 2020.

16. Thompson KA, Pappachan JV, Bennett AM, Mittal H, Macken S, Dove BK, et al. Influenza aerosols in UK hospitals during the H1N1 (2009) pandemic—the risk of aerosol generation during medical procedures. PLoS One 2013;8:e56278.

17. Tran K, Cimon K, Severn M, Pessoa-Silva CL, Conly J. Aerosol generating procedures and risk of transmission of acute respiratory infections to healthcare workers: a systematic review. PLoS One 2012;7:e35797.

18. Bourouiba L. Turbulent gas clouds and respiratory pathogen emissions: potential implications for reducing transmission of COVID-19. JAMA 2020 Mar 26 [Epub ahead of print].

19. Smith AC, Thomas E, Snoswell CL, Haydon H, Mehrotra A, Clemensen J, et al. Telehealth for global

emergencies: implications for coronavirus disease 2019 (COVID-19). J Telemed Telecare 2020 Mar 20 [Epub ahead of print].

20. Cheng VCC, Wong SC, Chen JHK, Yip CCY, Chuang VWM, Tsang OTY, et al. Escalating infection control response to the rapidly evolving epidemiology of the Coronavirus disease 2019 (COVID-19) due to SARS-CoV-2 in Hong Kong. Infect Control Hosp Epidemiol 2020 Mar 5 [Epub ahead of print].

21. Jefferson T, Del Mar CB, Dooley L, Ferroni E, Al-Ansary LA, Bawazeer GA, et al. Physical interventions to interrupt or reduce the spread of respiratory viruses. The Cochrane Database of Systematic Reviews 2011, Issue 7. Art. No.:CD006207. DOI: 10.1002/14651858. CD006207.pub4.

22. Centers for Disease Control and Prevention. Understanding the difference. Available at: https://www.cdc.gov/niosh/ npptl/pdfs/ UnderstandDifferenceInfographic-508.pdf. Retrieved April 12, 2020.

Chapter 4

Susceptibility to infection and clinical manifestation

Dr. Soumya Ranjan Panda,

Assistant Professor, Department of Obstetrics and Gynecology, AIIMS, Mangalagiri, Andhra Pradesh

Abstract

There is no specific affinity of COVID-19 with Pregnant women, and they do not appear more likely to be susceptible than the general population. The most common symptoms in pregnant women are only mild or moderate cold/flu-like symptoms. However, cough, fever, shortness of breath, headache and anosmia are also other relevant symptoms. Severe infection in pregnant women can present in the same way as the general population and early diagnosis, assessment and advocation of prompt supportive treatment is the key for successful treatment. At present, there are currently no data regarding the risk of miscarriage or early pregnancy loss with COVID-19 infection. No evidence exists about the teratogenicity of the virus.

4.1 Effect of COVID19 on Maternal and Fetal Outcome

From the historical point of view, both SARS-CoV and MERS-CoV were known to be responsible for severe complications during pregnancy.[1] However, there is no specific affinity of COVID-19 with Pregnant women, and they do not appear more likely to be susceptible than the general population. Moreover, as pregnancy is an immune-compromised state, response to viral infections, in general, can have severe symptoms, and this fact holds for COVID-19.[2]

4.2 Clinical manifestations

There is evolving evidence within the general population that there could be a cohort of asymptomatic individuals or those with minor symptoms who are carrying the virus, although the prevalence is unknown. The most common presentation in pregnant women is only mild to moderate cold/flu-like symptoms. However, cough, fever, shortness of breath, headache and anosmia are also other relevant symptoms. [3] More severe symptoms which suggest pneumonia and marked hypoxia are widely described with COVID-19 in older people, the immunosuppressed and those with chronic conditions such as diabetes, cancer or chronic lung disease.[4] The symptoms of severe infection are no different in pregnant women, and early identification and assessment for prompt supportive treatment are key.

The most common symptoms of COVID 19 are fever and cough, with more than 80% of hospitalized patients presenting with these symptoms.[5] Chen et al. analyzed nine women diagnosed with COVID-19 during the third trimester of pregnancy.[1] In this small series, the clinical presentation was similar to that seen in nonpregnant adults, with fever in seven, cough in four, myalgia in three, and sore throat and malaise each in two women. Five had lymphopenia. All had pneumonia, but none required mechanical ventilation, and none died. All women had a caesarean delivery, and APGARs were 8-9 at 1 minute and 9-10 at 5 minutes. Similarly, in their study, Zhu et al. analyzed another nine pregnancies with ten infants (one set of twins).[6] Clinical presentation of COVID-19 was similar to that seen in nonpregnant patients. Based on these limited reports, and the available data from other respiratory pathogens such as SARS and influenza, it is difficult to predict the clinical course of pregnant women with COVID-19. Hence the clinical course should be further evaluated in more number of well-designed follow-up studies in pregnant women and newborn babies.

More severe symptoms such as pneumonia and significant hypoxia are widely described with COVID-19 in older people, the immunosuppressed and those with other comorbid conditions such as diabetes, cancer and chronic lung disease. [7] These same symptoms can be a feature in pregnant women too. According to the Intensive Care National Audit and Research Centre in the UK report, out of the first 775 patients that were admitted to critical care settings with a diagnosis of COVID-19, five were pregnant.[3] Other reported cases of COVID-19 pneumonia in pregnancy are milder and with good recovery.[4]

4.3 Effects of COVID-19 on mother's health

a) risk of venous thromboembolism (VTE)

b) pregnant women with associated comorbidities: can present with increased severity with increased severity of clinical manifestations

c) increased rate of instrumental/operative delivery

d) increased risk of domestic violence and mental health

4.4 Effects On Foetus

Early pregnancy loss

At present, there are currently no data regarding the risk of miscarriage or early pregnancy loss with COVID-19 infection. Experience with SARS and MERS does not demonstrate a convincing relationship between disease and increased risk of miscarriage or second-trimester loss.[8]

Vertical transmission and teratogenicity

No evidence exists about the teratogenicity of the virus. Although there is very recent evidence suggesting a probability of vertical transmission, the proportion of affected pregnancies and the significance to the neonate has yet to be defined.[9,10]

4.5 Conclusion

There is no specific affinity of COVID-19 with Pregnant women, and they do not appear more likely to be susceptible than the general population. More severe symptoms such as pneumonia and significant hypoxia are widely described with COVID-19 in older people, the immunosuppressed and those with other comorbid conditions such as diabetes, cancer and chronic lung disease. Pregnant women having other comorbid conditions should be screened out in their early pregnancy, and special attention should be provided to them as they are at high risk for developing severe COVID-19 disease.

4.6 References

1. Al-Tawfq JA. Middle East Respiratory Syndrome Coronavirus (MERS-CoV) and COVID-19 infection during pregnancy. Travel Med Infect Dis [Internet]. 2020; https://www.ncbi.nlm.nih.gov/ pmc/articles/ PMC7118624.

2. Coronavirus (COVID-19) Infection in Pregnancy [Internet]. London: Royal College of Obstetricians and Gynaecologists; 2020 [cited 8th April 2020]. Available from: https://www.rcog.org.uk/globalassets/documents/guidelines/2020-04-03-coronavirus-covid-19-infection-in-pregnancy.pdf

3. ICNARC report on COVID-19 in critical care. In: ICNARC, ed., 2020.

4. Liu D, Li L, Wu X, et al. Pregnancy and Perinatal Outcomes of Women With Coronavirus Disease (COVID-19) Pneumonia: A Preliminary Analysis. American Journal of Roentgenology 2020:1-6. doi: 10.2214/ AJR.20.23072.

5. Chen N, Zhou M, Dong X, et al. Epidemiological and clinical characteristics of 99 cases of 2019 novel coronavirus pneumonia in Wuhan, China: a descriptive study. Lancet. 2020.

6. Zhu H, Wang L, Fang C, et al. Clinical analysis of 10 neonates born to mothers with 2019-nCoV pneumonia. TranslPediatr 2020;9(1):51-60. doi: http://dx.doi.org/10.21037/tp.2020.02.06

7. Guan W-j, Ni Z-y, Hu Y, et al. Clinical Characteristics of Coronavirus Disease 2019 in China. New England Journal of Medicine 2020 doi: 10.1056/NEJMoa2002032

8. Zhang J, Wang Y, Chen L, et al. Clinical analysis of pregnancy in second and third trimesters complicated severe acute respiratory syndrome. Zhonghua Fu Chan Ke Za Zhi2003;38:516-20.

9. Dong L, Tian J, He S, et al. Possible Vertical Transmission of SARS-CoV-2 From an Infected Mother to Her Newborn. JAMA 2020 doi: 10.1001/jama.2020.4621

10. Zeng H, Xu C, Fan J, et al. Antibodies in Infants Born to Mothers With COVID-19 Pneumonia. JAMA 2020 doi: 10.1001/jama.2020.4861.

Chapter 5

Place of care: Special arrangement and availability of essential facilities

Dr. Soumya Ranjan Panda,

Assistant Professor, Department of Obstetrics and Gynecology, AIIMS, Mangalagiri, Andhra Pradesh

Abstract

Pregnant women should immediately be isolated in a single room for screening if they have symptoms suggestive of COVID-19. Movement of such patients throughout the facility should be kept in a limit. A designated tertiary care hospital with effective isolation facilities should be the place of management for any Suspected, probable or confirmed cases of COVID-19 infection. An effective isolation facility is essential for managing suspected/probable cases. Besides, confirmed cases should be addressed in a negative-pressure isolation room. A confirmed patient that is critically ill should be admitted to a negative-pressure isolation room in an ICU. Hospitals should have multidisciplinary expertise (team of a midwife, obstetrician, specialist in intensive care medicine, microbiologist, anaesthetist and neonatologist) to manage critically ill obstetric patients. Patients should be triaged and stratified into the following.

5.1 Introduction

As the pandemic continues, the foremost problem inpatient care is mixing up of COVID and non-COVID cases and thereby a further easy and quick spread of the infection. Therefore every hospital should adopt certain changes in their previous management protocol to limit the spread of the disease.

5.2 Place of care

Pregnant women should immediately be isolated in a single room for screening if they have symptoms suggestive of COVID-19. Movement of such patients throughout the facility should be kept in a limit. A designated tertiary care hospital with effective isolation facilities should be the place of management for any Suspected, probable or confirmed cases of COVID-19 infection. An effective isolation facility is essential for managing suspected/probable cases. Besides, confirmed cases should be addressed in a negative-pressure isolation room. A confirmed patient that is critically ill should be admitted to a negative-pressure isolation room in an ICU. [1,2] Delivery of pregnant women with confirmed COVID-19 infection must take place in a dedicated negative pressure operating room. Hospitals should have a dedicated negative pressure operating room facility and a dedicated neonatal negative pressure isolation room for newborns. Ideally, these rooms should be nearer to one another so that the movements of concerned personnel can be limited. There is a good possibility that close familial contacts may represent asymptomatic carrier state. Hence the movement of such persons should be limited to the facility. However, providing such services may not be feasible every time and everywhere, especially in areas with widespread local transmission of the pandemic.

5.3 Triage

Hospitals should have multidisciplinary expertise (team of a midwife, obstetrician, specialist in intensive care medicine, microbiologist, anaesthetist and neonatologist) to manage critically ill obstetric patients. Patients should be triaged and stratified into the following categories based on clinical evaluation.

- ✓ Mild (symptomatic patient with stable vitals)
- ✓ Severe (patients presenting with a resting oxygen saturation of ≤93%, respiration rate ≥30/min and arterial blood oxygen partial pressure (PaO2)/ oxygen concentration (FiO2) ≤300 mmHg) or
- ✓ Critical (signs of shock with organ failure, respiratory failure requiring mechanical ventilation or refractory hypoxemia requiring extra-corporal membrane oxygenation)

While treating pregnant women with COVID-19 infection, special consideration should be given to physiological adaptations in pregnancy.

5.4 Immediate implementation of appropriate IPC (Infection prevention and control) measures: [3]

Adoption of IPC measures is a crucial step in the management of COVID-19 pandemic. WHO guidance is also available and should be adopted. [3] At the first point of contact, IPC measures should be taken, and patients suspected for COVID-19 should be given a mask and directed to a separate area. At least 1 m distance should be maintained between suspected patients. Standard precautions should be the norm in all areas of health care facilities. Personal Protective Equipment (respirator, goggle, face protective shield, surgical gown and gloves) should be donned by all attending medical staff when providing care for confirmed cases of COVID-19 infection. [4]

5.5 Current recommendations

FOGSI, in its good clinical practice recommendation on "pregnancy with covid-19 infection", has suggested some recommendations regarding arrangements in existing healthcare facilities to manage pregnant women with COVID-19 infection.[5] The salient points are-

- ✓ To minimise the risk of transmission, ideally, the management of COVID-19 exposed or infected pregnant women would be carried out in a unit dedicated only for managing COVID-19 exposed or infected pregnant women.

- ✓ Three separate zones should be demarcated in this unit, i.e. a) clean, b) potentially contaminated and c) contaminated.

- ✓ There should be an existence of exclusive passage to these three separate zones.
- ✓ In each of these zones, there should be a facility to deal with outpatient, inpatient care and intensive care management.
- ✓ Ideally, the entire contaminated zone (wards, labour rooms, operation theatres and ICU) should have a negative pressure system to contain the spread of infection.

However, providing such services may not be feasible every time and everywhere, especially in areas with widespread local transmission of the pandemic. But these principles can be applied to the existing facilities as far as possible to create an set up that close to ideal. The objective is to minimise the exposure of infectious patients by reducing the chance of contact between infected and non-infected pregnant women.

5.6 References

1. Diagnosis and treatment guideline for COVID-19 infection (trial version 6) [National Health Commission of the People's Republic of China website]. http://www.nhc.gov.cn. Accessed 18th March, 2020. [in Chinese]
2. The Lancet. Emerging understandings of 2019-nCoV. Lancet 2020; 395: 311.
3. Clinical management of severe acute respiratory infection (SARI) when COVID-19 disease is suspected Interim guidance 13th March 2020 [Internet]. Geneva: World Health Organization; 2020 [cited 7 April 2020].

Available from: https://www.who.int/docs/default-source/coronaviruse/clinical-management-of-novel-cov.pdf

4. Maxwell C, McGeer A, Tai KFY, Sermer M. No. 225 - Management guidelines for obstetric patients and neonates born to mothers with suspected or probable severe acute respiratory syndrome (SARS). J ObstetGynaecol Can 2017; 39: e130–e137.

5. [Internet]. Fogsi.org. 2020 [cited 24 September 2020]. Available from: https://www.fogsi.org/wp-content/uploads/covid19/fogsi_gcpr_on_pregnancy_with_COVID_19_version_2.pdf

Chapter 6

Antepartum, Intrapartum and Postpartum Care during COVID-19 pandemic.

Dr. Soumya Ranjan Panda,

Assistant Professor, Department of Obstetrics and Gynecology, AIIMS, Mangalagiri, Andhra Pradesh

The protocols of antepartum visit and care are based on years of evidence-based medicine and experience and hence should not be ignored. Most common clinical manifestations are fever, fatigue, myalgia, dry cough, and shortness of breath. Detection of viral nucleic acid using real-time polymerase chain reaction (RT-PCR) is considered the gold standard for the diagnosis. A chest Computed tomography scan (CT scan) without contrast is considered as one of the most useful investigations in clinical practice as it helps to confirm or rule out viral pneumonia and should be performed as clinically indicated. Growth scans during the antenatal period should be kept to a minimum and be performed only if clinically indicated. Patients infected with SARS-COV-2 are at an increased risk of developing both venous and arterial thromboembolism. Until there is an indication of urgent delivery based on the woman's respiratory condition, there is currently no evidence to favour one way of birth over another. Women with suspected, probable, or confirmed COVID-19 should continue to feed the newborn according to standard infant feeding guidelines.

6.1 Introduction

The high infectivity of the SARS-COV-2 and the inflicted lockdown and home quarantine has rendered people to remain at home. On the other hand, the protocols of antepartum visit and care are based on years of evidence-based medicine and experience and hence should not be ignored. As the current COVID-19 pandemic creates a situation of confusion, there is a high chance that some of the pregnant women may go on to miss some essential care. This may lead to unnecessary maternal sufferings. So caretakers should be very cautious to stress on essential visits.

6.2 Diagnosis

During the COVID-19 epidemic period, while attending pregnant patients even for routine care, a detailed history should be obtained, which must include the following points.

a) recent travel b) occupation c) significant contact and cluster and d) clinical manifestations

Case definition

For case definitions, we have used those definitions used by WHO's interim guidance, 'Global surveillance for COVID-19 disease caused by human infection with the 2019 novel coronavirus'.[1] WHO periodically updates the Global

Surveillance for human infection with coronavirus disease (COVID-19) document, which includes case definitions.

Suspect case

A. A patient having fever and at least one sign/symptom of respiratory disease, e.g., cough, shortness of breath (with acute respiratory illness), AND a history of residence or travel to a location reporting community transmission of COVID-19 disease during the preceding 14 days period of onset of symptoms; OR

B. A patient with any symptoms of acute respiratory illness AND coming in contact with a confirmed or probable COVID-19 case (see definition of contact) during the preceding 14 days period of onset of symptoms; OR

C. A patient having fever and at least one sign/symptom of respiratory disease, e.g., cough, shortness of breath (with acute respiratory illness); AND requiring hospitalization AND without having an alternative diagnosis that thoroughly explains the clinical presentation.

Probable case

A. A suspect case for whom COVID-19 testing gives an inconclusive result. OR

B. A suspect case for whom COVID-19 testing could not be performed for any reason.

Confirmed case

A person with confirmation of COVID-19 infection as on laboratory report with or without clinical signs and symptoms.

Clinical syndromes associated with COVID - 19 infections.

1. Mild illness
2. Pneumonia
3. Severe pneumonia
4. Acute respiratory distress syndrome
5. Sepsis
6. Septic shock

Most common clinical manifestations are fever, fatigue, myalgia, dry cough, and shortness of breath. Some may present with nasal congestion, runny nose, sore throat, haemoptysis, or diarrhoea. Peripheral white blood cells count can be normal or decreased in the early stages, and the lymphocyte count may be reduced. C-reactive protein may be increased. Some patients may have findings of mild thrombocytopenia, elevated levels of liver enzymes and creatinine phosphokinase.

Detection of viral nucleic acid using real-time polymerase chain reaction (RT-PCR) is considered the gold standard for the diagnosis. Specimens should be obtained primarily from the upper respiratory tract (nasopharyngeal and oropharyngeal swabs), lower respiratory tract(sputum, endotracheal aspirate, or bronchoalveolar lavage) and saliva. Repeat testing may be needed to confirm the diagnosis. If the viral nucleic acid from respiratory tract samples is not found on two separate occasions at least 24 hours apart, the diagnosis of COVID-19 can be ruled out.

A chest Computed tomography scan (CT scan) without contrast is considered as one of the most useful investigations in clinical practice as it helps to confirm or rule out viral pneumonia and should be performed as clinically indicated. A recent report found the sensitivity of chest CT in diagnosing COVID-19 to be greater than that of RT-PCR (98% vs 71%). [2]

6.3. Management

Management algorithm for management of COVID-19 patients with pregnancy is shown in figure-1.

6.3.A. *Antenatal care*

As the majority of antenatal and postnatal care are regarded as essential care, women should be encouraged to attend the same as long as they do not meet criteria of current self-isolation guidance.[3-5] While attending for routine antenatal visits, they should adopt social distancing measures and personal hygiene. A group of clinicians should be dedicated to coordinate care for women forced to miss appointments due to self-isolation.

Women should be able to notify the hospital about their self-isolation through telephone numbers that should be provided to them by the hospital. Appointments should then be fixed based on need or urgency.[6]

For women who have symptoms, appointments can be deferred until seven days from the onset of symptoms, unless the symptoms (aside from persistent cough) persevere. Similarly, appointments should be deferred for 14 days, for those who are self-isolating because someone in their household has possible symptoms of COVID-19. Hospitals should monitor serial appointments, and any missed appointment should be noted.

Arrangements should be made to contact those women whose routine appointment is delayed for more than three weeks.[7]

Although available research is insufficient to estimate the effects of smoking, manifestations of COVID-19 may likely get worsened. Hence emphasis should be given to stop smoking for all women who do.[8]

6.3.B. *Antenatal Growth scans*

Growth scans during the antenatal period should be kept to a minimum and be performed only if clinically indicated. However, a foetal growth scan should be performed in women who have been diagnosed with severe or critical disease. According to RCOG, this scan should be offered approximately 14 days after recovery from the viral illness, unless an earlier scan is indicated for any pre-existing clinical reason (e.g. foetal growth restriction).[9]

6.3.C. *Thromboprophylaxis*

Patients infected with SARS-COV-2 are at an increased risk of developing both venous and arterial thromboembolism. This has been attributed to excessive inflammation, hypoxia, immobilization and intravascular coagulation.[10] Recent studies have found an incidence of 25% to 31% of venous or arterial thromboembolism in admitted patients with COVID-19.[10,11] At the same time, pregnancy itself is a hypercoagulable state. Hence there exists a risk of aggravation of thrombotic state in pregnant women affected with COVID-19. Various guidelines, including RCOG, recommend thromboprophylaxis on an individualized basis for women with high-risk factors for venous thromboembolism who are advised for self-isolation.[9,12] As per the RCOG recommendation, all pregnant women admitted with confirmed or suspected COVID-19 disease should receive a prophylactic dose of Low Molecular Weight Heparin (LMWH) unless birth is expected within 12 hours.[9] For high-risk patients, a haematological consultation may be needed for any increase in dose or duration of prophylaxis.

FIGURE-1: Flow chart showing management of obstetrics patients during COVID-19 pandemic

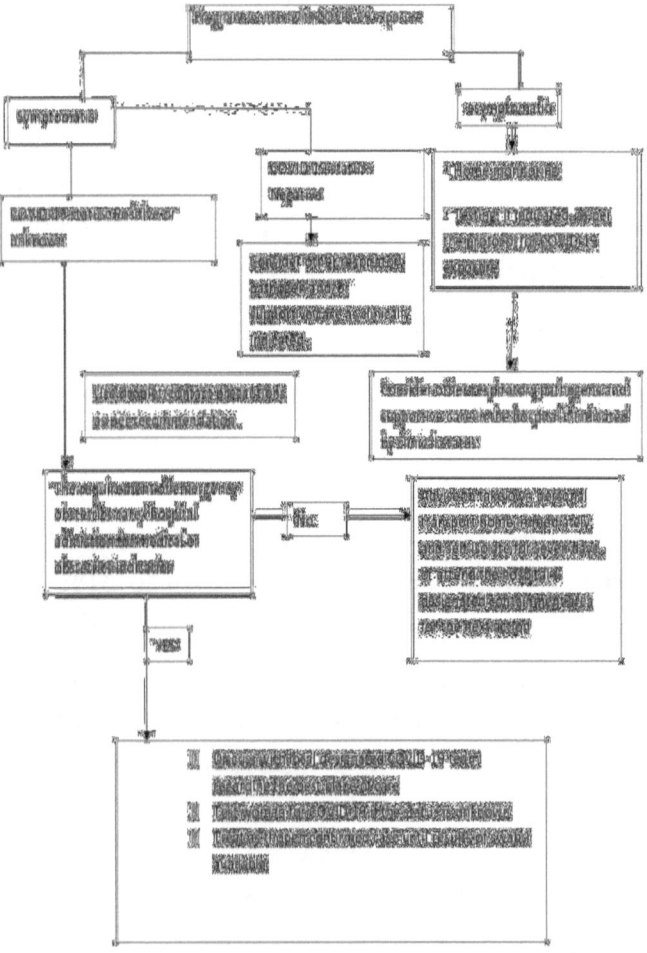

6.3.D. Intrapartum care for patients with suspected or confirmed COVID-19

- Assessment of the severity of COVID-19 symptoms by a multidisciplinary team (MDT), including infectious diseases or general medical specialist.
- Observation of maternal vitals including temperature, respiratory rate and oxygen saturation.
- Onset of labour should be confirmed as per standard care.

6.3.E. Fetal surveillance during labour

At present, foetal monitoring of asymptomatic pregnant women is not recommended. However, continuous Electronic foetal monitoring should be recommended for all symptomatic patients in labour.[9]

6.3.F. Tocolysis for preterm labour

For woman infected with COVID-19 and presenting with spontaneous preterm labour, tocolysis should not be attempted to delay delivery to administer antenatal steroids.[13]

6.3.G. Steroid use for lung maturation

Provided availability of adequate childbirth and newborn care, WHO and ISUOG guidelines recommend administration of antenatal corticosteroid for women at risk of preterm birth between 24 to 34 weeks of gestation if no clinical evidence of maternal infection could be found out. However, for women with mild COVID-19, the clinical benefits of antenatal corticosteroid might outweigh the risks of potential harm to the mother. In these conditions, the clinical condition of the woman, the benefits and harms related to corticosteroids should be discussed with the woman and other family members to ensure an informed decision.[9,14]

6.3.H. Elective induction of labour

Although the results of a recent randomized controlled trial comparing induction of labour with expectant management (ARRIVE), showed that the caesarean section rate was not increased with induction at 39 weeks, it did highlight that there was an increase in time to delivery and length of stay.[15] Thus there appears an increased risk of exposure for both patients and staff. Hence, we opine that elective inductions, especially when accompanied by a poor bishop's score, should be postponed. However, this recommendation does not hold true for medically or obstetrically indicated inductions.

6.3.I. Mode of delivery

Unless the woman's respiratory condition demands urgent delivery, there is currently no evidence to favour one way of birth over another. Therefore, the mode of birth should be decided based upon any obstetric indications for intervention and her preferences, and it should not be influenced by mere presence or absence of COVID-19.[16] At present, a lack of evidence to find the presence of SARS-COV-2 in vaginal secretions.

In the case of Septic shock, acute organ failure or foetal distress decision for prompt emergency Caesarean delivery (or termination) can be taken.[13,17] At present water birth should be avoided as a safety concern for health personnel. [13,16]

6.3.J. Shortening of the Second stage of labour

A prolonged second stage may culminate in an increased risk of respiratory secretion exposures to visitors and medical personnel.[18] Hence some authors are in a view to resume previous recommendations, i.e. to allow a 1-hour second stage duration in a multiparous patient without an epidural (or 2 hours with an epidural) and a 2-hour second stage duration in a nulliparous patient without an epidural (or 3 hours with an epidural). [19] At present RCOG and ISUOG guidelines recommend cutting short the second stage with an operative vaginal delivery in symptomatic patients those become exhausted and hypoxic. [9,13]

6.3.K. Anaesthesia

Again, there is a lack of evidence for preferring any particular type of anaesthesia (epidural or spinal analgesia or anaesthesia). Hence to minimize the requirement of general anaesthesia if urgent delivery is needed, epidural analgesia should be preferred in labour, in women with suspected or confirmed COVID-19.[13,16]

6.3.L. Cord clamping

Keeping an eye on the beneficial effects and a lack of evidence for transmission of the virus in cord blood, the current recommendation should be delayed cord clamping following birth, unless contraindicated. The baby should be cleaned and dried as usual, while the cord is still intact.[16]

6.3.M. Breastfeeding

Women with suspected, probable, or confirmed COVID-19 should continue to feed the newborn according to standard infant feeding guidelines. Infection prevention and control (IPC), as appropriate, should be adopted while breastfeeding. Practise of respiratory hygiene and hand hygiene is of utmost importance for all confirmed, suspected COVID-19 cases or symptomatic mothers who are breastfeeding or practising skin-to-skin contact or kangaroo mother care. They should be advised to practice these hygiene measures before and after contact with the child. Also, they should be advised to routinely clean and disinfect surfaces with which the symptomatic mother has been in contact. Critically ill women with COVID-19 or those with other complications that prevent her from continuing breastfeeding should be supported to express milk, and safely provide breast milk to the infant while applying appropriate IPC measures.[14]

6.3.N. Abortus (embryos, foetuses and placentae)

of COVID-19-infected women should be treated as potentially infectious tissues, and there should be the availability of the appropriate and safe disposal facility. if possible, testing of these tissues for COVID-19 by qRT-PCR should be undertaken.[13]

6.4 Management pregnant women with COVID-19 with severe/ critical illness

6.4.A. Supportive therapy

It is essential to advice adequate rest, nutritional support and water and electrolyte balance. Hydration should be maintained.

Maternal observation with close monitoring of vital signs and oxygen saturation remains the cornerstone of supportive care. Based on the degree of hypoxemia supplemental oxygen inhalation (60%-100% concentration at a rate of 5 L/min) can be given via high-flow nasal cannula. Oxygenation can be maintained by intubation, mechanical ventilation or even extra-corporal membrane oxygenation (ECMO). As infection with SARS-COV-2 can culminate in complications like septic shock, acute kidney injury, and virus-induced cardiac injury, it is essential to monitor arterial blood gases, renal function, liver function, serum lactate level and cardiac enzymes as indicated by the clinical situation. A chest computed tomography scan (CT scan) without contrast is considered as one of the most useful investigations in clinical practice as it helps to confirm or rule out viral pneumonia and should be performed as clinically indicated.

6.4.B. Fluid management

Conservative fluid management measures should be adopted for critically ill patients without shock.[17] Those with septic shock should be managed with volume resuscitation and norepinephrine to maintain mean arterial blood pressure (MAP) at the level of 60 mm Hg or above. [20] Hourly fluid input/output charts should be used in managing women with moderate to severe COVID-19 cases, keeping in mind the fact that these cases can worsen as respiratory distress and failure. Thus, every effort should be made to target a neutral fluid balance in labour to avoid the risk of fluid overload.[16]

6.4.C. Oxygenation

To maintain adequate foetal oxygenation, an SpO2 of 95% and above should be maintained for pregnant women. [21,22] Immediate Oxygen therapy is necessary to prevent hypoxemia and reduce the work of breathing. High-flow or non-rebreather mask may be used for oxygen delivery according to the patient's clinical condition. Humidification therapy devices, non-invasive ventilation (NIV), or endotracheal intubation may be necessary.[23-26] Of late, the use of extracorporeal membrane lung oxygenation technology (ECMO) has been indicated to reduce the death of patients with pulmonary infection. [27-30] Nevertheless, during pregnancy, its use should be limited and less invasive therapy initiated early, to prevent and treat severe respiratory complications.[26]

6.4.D. Antiviral treatment

Although clinical trials involving various drugs are undergoing, currently, there is no proven antiviral treatment for COVID-19 patients. Antiretroviral drugs are being trialled therapeutically on patients with severe symptoms.[15,17] As advised by WHO caution and careful risk-benefit analysis should be exercised before using investigational therapeutic agents in pregnant women outside clinical trials. Remdesivir (a nucleotide analogue), chloroquine (an antimalarial drug) and hydroxychloroquine are some of the drugs against COVID-19 that found to inhibit SARS-COV-2 virus in vitro.[31]

6.4.E. Antibiotic treatment

The extensive lung damage by the virus leads to a substantially increased risk of secondary bacterial pneumonia. Antibiotic treatment is indicated if there is evidence of secondary bacterial infection. However, antibiotic administration should not be delayed if bacterial sepsis is suspected. Antibiotics can be initiated to ensure broad-spectrum coverage for women with suspected or confirmed secondary bacterial infections. Antibiotics should be tailored to drug sensitivity results.[32]

6.4.F. Corticosteroid therapy

Outside clinical trials, systemic corticosteroids for the treatment of viral pneumonia should not be routinely used.[14]

Severe acute renal failure due to sepsis: haemodialysis may be required should severe sepsis lead to renal failure, and should electrolyte imbalances be so impaired that they are life-threatening and unresponsive to conservative management.

6.5 Summary

A. It appears that pregnant women bear the same risk of getting an infection as the general population. However, as pregnancy is an immune-compromised state, response to viral infections, in general, can have severe symptoms.

B. Viral nucleic acid detection of SARS-COV-2 using real-time polymerase chain reaction (RT-PCR) is considered the gold standard for the diagnosis of COVID-19.

C. Radiological evaluations like X-ray or computed tomography (CT) scan of the chest without contrast are considered as valuable investigations as these help to confirm or rule out viral pneumonia and should be performed as clinically indicated.

D. A designated tertiary care hospital with adequate isolation facilities should be the place of management for any Suspected, probable or confirmed cases of COVID-19 infection. A Suspected or probable case during pregnancy should be managed in isolation, and confirmed cases should be addressed in a negative-pressure isolation room. A confirmed case that is critically ill should be admitted to a negative-pressure isolation room in an ICU

E. Personal Protective Equipment (respirator, goggle, face protective shield, surgical gown and gloves) should be donned by all attending medical staff when providing care for confirmed cases of COVID-19 infection.

F. Hospitals should have multidisciplinary expertise (team of a midwife, obstetrician, specialist in intensive care medicine, microbiologist, anaesthetist and neonatologist) to manage critically ill obstetric patients. Patients should be triaged and stratified into a mild, severe and critical category for better management.

G. The majority of care planned for antenatal and postnatal women is considered as essential care, and hence, women should be encouraged to attend the same.

H. While attending for routine antenatal visits, they should adopt social distancing measures and personal hygiene.

I. Continuous Electronic fetal monitoring should be recommended for all women with COVID-19 in labour.

J. For woman infected with COVID-19 and presenting with spontaneous preterm labour, tocolysis should not be attempted to delay delivery in order to administer antenatal steroids.

K. Caution should be exercised while using antenatal steroids (dexamethasone or betamethasone) for fetal lung maturation in a critically ill patient. However, antenatal corticosteroid therapy can be advised for women at risk of preterm birth between 24 to 34 weeks of gestation if there is no clinical evidence of maternal infection.

L. Unless there is a need for urgent delivery due to woman's respiratory condition, currently no evidence exists to favour one way of birth over another.

M. To minimize the requirement of general anaesthesia if urgent delivery is needed, epidural analgesia should be preferred in labour, in women with suspected or confirmed COVID-19.

N. Cord clamping: Given a lack of evidence for transmission of the virus in cord blood, the current recommendation should be delayed cord clamping following birth provided there are no other contraindications.

O. Women with suspected, probable, or confirmed COVID-19 should continue to feed the newborn according to standard infant feeding guidelines. Infection prevention and control (IPC), as appropriate, should be adopted while breastfeeding.

P. Outside clinical trials, systemic corticosteroids for the treatment of viral pneumonia should not be routinely used.

6.6 References

1. Global surveillance for COVID-19 caused by human infection with COVID-19 virus Interim guidance 20th March 2020 [Internet]. Geneva: World Health Organization; 2020 [cited 7 April 2020]. Available from: https://apps.who.int/iris/rest/bitstreams/1272502/retrieve

2. Ai T, Yang Z, Hou H, et al. Correlation of chest CT and RT-PCR testing in Coronavirus Disease 2019 (COVID-19) in China: a report of 1014 cases. Radiology. 2020. https://doi.org/10.1148/radiol.20202 00642

3. Stay at home: guidance for households with possible coronavirus (COVID-19) infection 2020 [Available from: https://www.gov.uk/government/publications/covid-19-stay-at-home-guidance/stay-at-home-guidancefor-households-with-possible-coronavirus-covid-19-infection accessed 17th March 2020.

4. Major new measures to protect people at highest risk from coronavirus 2020 [Available from: https://www. gov.uk/government/news/major-new-measures-to-protect-people-at-highest-risk-from-coronavirus accessed 26 March 2020.

5. Dowswell T, Carroli G, Duley L, et al. Alternative versus standard packages of antenatal care for low-risk pregnancy. Cochrane Database of Systematic Reviews 2015(7) doi: 10.1002/14651858.CD000934.pub3

6. COVID-19: guidance on social distancing and for vulnerable people 2020 [Available from: https://www.

gov. uk/government/publications/covid-19-guidance-on-social-distancing-and-for-vulnerable-people accessed 17 March 2020.

7. Coronavirus (COVID-19) Infection in Pregnancy [Internet]. London; 2020 [cited 6 April 2020]. Available from: https://www.rcog.org.uk/globalassets/documents/guidelines/2020-04-03-coronavirus-covid-19-infection-in-pregnancy.pdf

8. Vardavas CI, Nikitara K. COVID-19 and smoking: A systematic review of the evidence. Tobacco Induced Diseases 2020;18(March) doi: 10.18332/tid/119324

9. 9.Rcog.org.uk.2020.[online]Availableat:<https://www.rcog.org.uk/globalassets/documents/guidelines/2020-07-24-coronavirus-covid-19-infection-in-pregnancy.pdf> [Accessed 15 September 2020].

10. Klok FA, Kruip MJHA, van der Meer NJM *et al* Incidence of thrombotic complications in critically ill ICU patients with COVID-19. Thromb Res. 2020: S0049-3848 (20): 30120-110.1016/j.thromres.2020.04.013. [PMC free article] [PubMed] [CrossRef] [Google Scholar]

11. Cui S, Chen S, Li X, Liu S, Wang F. Prevalence of venous thromboembolism in patients with severe novel coronavirus pneumonia. J ThrombHaemost. 2020. 10.1111/jth.14830, 10.1111/jth.14830. [PMC free article] [PubMed] [CrossRef] [CrossRef] [Google Scholar]

12. RCPI IoOaG . COVID-19 Infection Guidance for Maternity Services. Version 3.0. 2020. Available from

URL: https://www.rcpi.ie/news/releases/theinstitute-of-obstetricians-and-gynaecologists-issuesguidance-on-covid-19-and-maternity-services/.

13. Poon L, Yang H, Lee J, Copel J, Leung T, Zhang Y et al. ISUOG Interim Guidance on 2019 novel coronavirus infection during pregnancy and puerperium: information for healthcare professionals. Ultrasound in Obstetrics &Gynecology [Internet]. 2020 [cited 7 April 2020];. Available from: https://obgyn.onlinelibrary.wiley.com/doi/10.1002/uog.22013

14. Clinical management of severe acute respiratory infection (SARI) when COVID-19 disease is suspected Interim guidance 13th March 2020 [Internet]. Geneva: World Health Organization; 2020 [cited 7 April 2020]. Available from: https://www.who.int/docs/default-source/coronaviruse/clinical-management-of-novel-cov.pdf

15. Grobman WA, Rice MM, Reddy UM, et al; Eunice Kennedy Shriver National Institute of Child Health and Human Development Maternal–Fetal Medicine Units Network. Labor induction versus expectant management in low-risk nulliparous women. N Engl J Med 2018;379(06):513–523

16. Zhu H, Wang L, Fang C, et al. Clinical analysis of 10 neonates born to mothers with 2019-nCoV pneumonia. TranslPediatr 2020;9(1):51-60. doi: http://dx.doi.org/10.21037/tp.2020.02.06

17. American College of Radiology. ACR-SPR practice parameter for imaging pregnant or potentially pregnant

adolescents and women with ionizing radiation. Revised 2018. https://www.acr.org/-/media/ACR/Files/Practice-Parameters/Pregnant-Pts.pdf

18. Caughey AB, Cahill AG, Guise JM, Rouse DJ; American College of Obstetricians and Gynecologists (College); Society for MaternalFetal Medicine. Safe prevention of the primary cesarean delivery. Am J ObstetGynecol 2014;210(03):179–193

19. Stephens A, Barton J, Bentum N, Blackwell S, Sibai B. General Guidelines in the Management of an Obstetrical Patient on the Labor and Delivery Unit during the COVID-19 Pandemic. American Journal of Perinatology. 2020;37(08):829-836.

20. Committee Opinion No. 723: Guidelines for diagnostic imaging during pregnancy and lactation. ObstetGynecol 2017; 130: e210–e216.

21. The Lancet. Emerging understandings of 2019-nCoV. Lancet 2020; 395: 311.

22. Tremblay E, Therasse E, Thomassin-Naggara I, Trop I. Quality initiatives: guidelines' for use of medical imaging during pregnancy and lactation. Radiographics 2012; 32: 897–911.

23. Centers for Disease Control. Interim Clinical Guidance for Management of Patients with Confirmed Coronavirus Disease (COVID-19). https://www.cdc.gov/ coronavirus/2019-ncov/hcp/clinical-guidance-management-patients.html [Accessed 8th March 2020].

24. Boseley S. China trials anti-HIV drug on coronavirus patients. The Guardian [cited 15th February 2020]. https://www.theguardian.com/world/2020/feb/07/china-trials-antihiv-drug-coronavirus-patients.

25. NIH clinical trial of remdesivir to treat COVID-19 begins. 25th February 2020. https://www.nih.gov/news-events/news-releases/nih-clinical-trial-remdesivir-treatcovid-19-begins [Accessed 9 March 2020].

26. Metlay JP, Waterer GW, Long AC, Anzueto A, Brozek J, Crothers K et al.; on behalf of the American Thoracic Society and Infectious Diseases Society of America. Diagnosis and Treatment of Adults with Community-acquired Pneumonia. An Official Clinical Practice Guideline of the American Thoracic Society and Infectious Diseases Society of America. Am J Respir Crit Care Med 2019; 200: e45–e67.

27. 27.49. Rasmussen SA, Smulian JC, Lednicky JA, Wen TS, Jamieson DJ. Coronavirus Disease 2019 (COVID-19) and pregnancy: what obstetricians need to know. Am J ObstetGynecol 2020. DOI: 10.1016/j.ajog.2020.02.017.

28. 28.50. Schultz MJ, Dunser MW, Dondorp AM, Adhikari NKJ, Iyer S, Kwizera A, Lubell Y, Papali A, Pisani L, Riviello ED, Angus DC, Azevedo LC, Baker T, Diaz JV, Festic E, et al. Current challenges in the management of sepsis in ICUs in resource-poor settings and suggestions for the future. Intensive Care Med 2017; 43: 612–624.

29. Plante LA, Pacheco LD, Louis JM. SMFM Consult Series #47: Sepsis during pregnancy and the puerperium. Am J ObstetGynecol 2019; 220: B2–B10.

30. Røsjø H, Varpula M, Hagve TA, Karlsson S, Ruokonen E, Pettila V, Omland T; FINNESEPSIS Study Group. Circulating high sensitivity troponin T in severe sepsis and septic shock: distribution, associated factors, and relation to outcome. Intensive Care Med 2011; 37: 77–85.

31. Wang M, Cao R, Zhang L, et al. Remdesivir and chloroquine effectively inhibit the recently emerged novel coronavirus (2019- nCoV) in vitro. Cell Res. 2020. https://doi.org/10.1038/s4142 2-020-0282-0

32. Miller RW. Discussion: severe mental retardation and cancer among atomic bomb survivors exposed in utero. Teratology 1999; 59: 234–235.

Chapter 7

Contraceptive advice and reproductive health care during COVID-19 pandemic.

Dr. Soumya Ranjan Panda,

Assistant Professor, Department of Obstetrics and Gynecology, AIIMS, Mangalagiri, Andhra Pradesh

Abstract

Contraception appears to be lifesaving and an essential component of reproductive health care in that it improves women's reproductive autonomy and reduces unintended pregnancies. As medical communities prepare to tackle the current pandemic, strategies to mitigate virus spread and optimise health care resources are evolving and will need to be country-specific. Thus, while elective surgeries and non-urgent appointments are getting cancelled, health care providers should strive to ensure continuity of reproductive health care to women which have the ability to reduce maternal and infant mortality. Telemedicine facilities should be used to screen, counsel, prescribe, and manage complications related to oral contraceptives. Abortion is an essential component of comprehensive health care, and it is no recommended that COVID-19 responses should cancel or delay abortion procedures.

7.1 Background

Unintended pregnancies count for approximately 50% of the cause.[1] Especially in low- and middle-income countries, where access to health care may be limited, this can have a grave consequence leading to unsafe abortion or other serious pregnancy complications that contribute to maternal and infant mortality.[2] Thus, contraception appears to be lifesaving and an essential component of reproductive health care in that it improves women's reproductive autonomy and reduces unintended pregnancies. However, the major obstacles in the use of contraception are its availability, accessibility and lack of motivation to use.

As medical communities prepare to tackle the current pandemic, strategies to mitigate virus spread and optimise health care resources are evolving and will need to be country-specific. Thus, while elective surgeries and non-urgent appointments are getting cancelled, health care providers should strive to ensure continuity of reproductive health care to women which have the ability to reduce maternal and infant mortality. At the same time, one should be careful to minimise unnecessary hospital visits to reduce the exposure to SARS-COV-2.

7.2 Selected strategies for improving contraception access during the COVID-19 pandemic

According to ACOG recommendation, telemedicine facilities should be used to screen, counsel, prescribe, and manage complications related to oral contraceptives. They recommend refilling contraceptives for the full year, and providing advance prescriptions for emergency contraception, if necessary. Wherever possible, long-acting reversible contraceptives (LARC) like the insertion of IUDs or contraceptive implants, and permanent contraception should be offered. Oral contraceptives can be advised If LARC methods are unavailable, as a bridge to delayed insertion. Of note, ACOG also recommends postponing routine LARC removals, if possible. This is due to the fact that there is demonstrable effectiveness of extended use of IUDs beyond the labelled duration. Furthermore, clinical trial data support the extended use of LARC devices beyond approved durations. For example, the effectiveness of copper T380A, the 52 mg levonorgestrel IUD and the etonogestrel implant remains for 12 years, seven years and five years of use respectively. ACOG also supports the advantage of over-the-counter hormonal contraception programs in states/ regions where this practice is allowed.[3]

With regard to abortion, ACOG, along with American Society for Reproductive Medicine (ASRM) and the Society of Family Planning (SFM), in their joint statement addressed that abortion is an essential component of comprehensive health care and do not support COVID-19 responses that cancel or delay abortion procedures. As abortion is a time-sensitive service for which a delay of several days or weeks can potentially make it completely inaccessible and in turn can have grave consequences which can profoundly impact a person's life, health, and well-being. It also states to have collaboration between community-based and hospital-based clinicians to ensure abortion access is not compromised during this period. [4] A "no-test" protocol, is recommended which allows patients at <77 days of gestation to have access evidence-based, safe medication abortion without in-person visits. The treatment package includes mifepristone, misoprostol, ibuprofen, and/or post-abortion contraception.[5]

SFM recommendations are also quite similar to ACOG recommendations with few additional measures. SFM recommends that oral contraceptive advice should not be withheld for lack of blood pressure or BMI documentation. Patients can be advised to check their blood pressure using a purchased cuff at home. However, if one is not available, they recommend prescribing contraceptives after counselling patients of the risks. With regard to depot-medroxyprogesterone acetate (DMPA) injections, they recommend considering a prescription for the subcutaneous formulation, which can be self-administered. They also recommend maintaining access to postpartum tubal ligation.[6]

WHO recommends countries develop innovative strategies to ensure as many eligible people as possible can access information and contraception during this period by increasing the use of mobile phones and digital technologies. [7] In addition to expanding the availability of contraceptive resources in healthcare facilities, they recommend increasing information and access at pharmacies, drug shops, online platforms, and other outlets. With regard to emergency contraception, they support developing plans to increase access to emergency post-coital contraception, including consideration of over-the-counter provision. They recommend enabling access to contraception for women and girls in the immediate postpartum and post-abortion periods. Finally, they encourage health care workers to provide contraceptive information and services as per national guidelines to the full extent possible, particularly in areas where the pregnancy poses a high risk to health.[7]

Exercise plays a vital role in reproductive health. Measures taken to combat COVID19 pandemic may promote a sedentary lifestyle and thereby exacerbating another established global pandemic known as physical inactivity. Clinicians can help out their patients in promoting and proposing supportive lifestyle care. Even if we need to restrict ourselves indoor, care must be taken to spend more time in indoor physical activity and less time sitting.[8]

7.3 References

1. Bearak J, Popinchalk A, Alkema L, Sedgh G. Global, regional, and subregional trends in unintended pregnancy and its outcomes from 1990 to 2014: estimates from a Bayesian hierarchical model. Lancet Glob Health. 2018;6(4):e380–389. 10.1016/s2214-109x(18)30029-9. [PMC free article] [PubMed] [CrossRef] [Google Scholar]

2. World Bank. *Trends in Maternal Mortality 2000 to 2017: Estimates by WHO, UNICEF, UNFPA, World Bank Group and the United Nations Population Division (Vol. 2) (English)*. Washington, DC: World Bank Group; 2019. Accessed April 1, 2020 http://documents.

worldbank.org/curated/en/793971568908763231/Trends-in-maternal-mortality-2000-to-2017-Estimates-by-WHO-UNICEF-UNFPA-World-Bank-Group-and-the-United-Nations-Population-Division [Google Scholar]

3. COVID-19 FAQs for obstetricians-gynecologists, gynaecology. American College of Obstetricians and Gynecologists 2020; Available from: https://www.acog.org/clinical-.

4. Joint Statement on Abortion Access During the COVID-19 Outbreak. Washington: American college of obstetricians and gynecologists; 2020.

5. Raymond EG, et al. Commentary: no-test medication abortion: a sample protocol for increasing access during a pandemic and beyond. Contraception. 2020;101(6):361–366. doi: 10.1016/j.contraception.2020.04.005. [PMC free article] [PubMed] [CrossRef] [Google Scholar]

6. Benson LS, Madden T, Tarleton J. Society of Family Planning. 2020. Society of Family Planning interim clinical recommendations: Contraceptive provision when healthcare access is restricted due to pandemic response. [Google Scholar]

7. Stover J, Ross J. How increased contraceptive use has reduced maternal mortality. Matern Child Health J. 2010;14(5):687–695. doi: 10.1007/s10995-009-0505-y. [PubMed] [CrossRef] [Google Scholar]

8. Panda SR. Alliance of COVID 19 with pandemic of sedentary lifestyle & physical inactivity: Impact on

reproductive health. Taiwan J Obstet Gynecol. 2020 Sep;59(5):790. doi: 10.1016/j.tjog.2020.07.034. Epub 2020 Jul 15. PMID: 32917342; PMCID: PMC7362860.

Chapter 8

Laparoscopy and Hysteroscopy during COVID-19 pandemic

Dr. Soumya Ranjan Panda,

Assistant Professor, Department of Obstetrics and Gynecology, AIIMS, Mangalagiri, Andhra Pradesh

Abstract

The COVID-19 related morbidity and high mortality further increase significantly during peri and postoperative period. Surgery is considered as a high-risk situation for the transmission of respiratory infections. Most of the international societies advice deferral of elective surgery except for cancer surgeries and other emergency surgeries during this pandemic. SARS-COV-2 may be transmitted via droplets and fomites. Airborne transmission is described as another mode, whereby the virus can remain in the air for long periods within droplets. Highest transmission risk has been observed with medical and patient care activities that can result in the release of airborne particles (aerosols). Both ultrasonic and electrosurgical devices can create large surgical plumes. Hence both the energy devices can potentially increase the risks of viral transmission. Although both open and laparoscopic surgery has the potential to generate aerosols, the overall risk seems to be lower with laparotomies as there is no requirement of creation of an artificial pneumoperitoneum. Hence the present scenario demands the role of a clinician in balancing the hypothetical risk of aerosol spread in low-risk patients to already established evidence of benefits of laparoscopic surgery.

8.1 Background

COVID-19 pneumonia often requires hospitalisation and intensive care treatment. The COVID-19 related morbidity and high mortality further increase significantly during peri and postoperative period. Surgery is considered as a high-risk situation for the transmission of respiratory infections. [1] Therefore, it would be prudent to scrutinise and postpone any surgical treatment if possible. At the same time, however, women continue to require treatment for several gynecologic pathologies, some of which cannot be postponed. Nonsurgical, conservative treatment, including pharmacological therapies for hormone-sensitive pathologies, should be preferred over surgical treatment.

Hence most of the international societies advice deferral of elective surgery except for cancer surgeries and other emergency surgeries during this pandemic.[2-5] Conduction of endoscopic procedures have been more challenging during this pandemic as theoretically these procedures can put all involved personnel at increased risk of inhalation and conjunctival exposure from bioaerosol (endoscopically generated and otherwise).[6-10] So it is very much essential to review current practices that will help safe Conduction of such procedures.

8.2 General considerations

SARS-COV-2 may be transmitted via droplets and fomites. Airborne transmission is described as another mode, whereby the virus can remain in the air for long periods within droplets of size less than five μm in diameter and can later be transmitted to others over distances greater than one meter.[11] Airborne transmission is particularly important in specific circumstances that generate aerosols, such as endotracheal intubation, airway manipulation, and probably surgery.

The size of COVID-19 virion is approximately 0.125 mm and are most commonly transmitted as more massive (>20 mm) respiratory water droplets. The virus may be aerosolised and transmitted in smaller droplets as well.

In COVID-19 infected patients, the presence of the virus in the body cavity can lead to nebulisation in the spray generated by surgical instruments during surgery. Hence the aerosol generated in an operating room during surgery is capable of containing the virus or parts of it. Even it has been suggested by some authors that the virus can be viable in the aerosol for at least three hours.[12] However, there almost no evidence from the current pandemic or prior global influenza epidemics to conclude that respiratory viruses are transmitted via an aerosol generated in the operating room.

8.3 Viral transmission in surgically generated smoke and aerosols

8.3. A. Infection risk with SARS-CoV-2 in endoscopy/laparoscopy

During endoscopic procedures, the theoretical risk of infection related to bioaerosols might be increased due to the following three factors [13,14]

1. Pneumoperitoneum creation via CO2 insufflations.
2. Use of electrosurgery and
3. Inadvertent gas leaks.

Highest transmission risk has been observed with medical and patient care activities that can result in the release of airborne particles (aerosols). These aerosol-generating procedures (AGPs) can create a risk of airborne transmission of infections. Intubation and extubation are considered as one of the highest risk AGPs due to the presence of high viral load in respiratory secretions.[15]

An aerosol is a suspension system of solid or liquid particles in gas and includes both the particles and the suspending gas. The gaseous medium is usually air, and in the case of laparoscopy, it's CO2. Studies have shown that whole cells can be carried as aerosols in the pneumoperitoneum during laparoscopy in the smoke produced by cauterisation.[16, 17] It seems that increasing pneumoperitoneum pressure is directly proportional to the number of cells found. [18]

Recently, Mallick et al. in their review concluded a lack of evidence surrounding aerosolisation.[19] Studies have identified pathogens such as human papillomavirus (HPV), Corynebacterium, hepatitis B virus (HBV) and human immunodeficiency virus (HIV) in surgical smoke. Around 40 % of HPV during large loop excision of the transformation zone (LLETZ) procedures, while roughly 90 % of HBV during laparoscopies in infected patients have been documented. However, despite the high number of pathogens in smoke plumes, there is a very few actual reported cases of transmission, with four confirmed cases of HPV and none of HBV or HIV.

Although these facts are quite reassuring, caution should be maintained, especially when dealing with the potentially more virulent pathogens such as SARS-CoV-2. [6–10]

8.3.B. Energy modalities

As discussed, both ultrasonic and electrosurgical devices can create large surgical plumes. Hence both the energy devices can potentially increase the risks of viral transmission. As stated by NHS pandemic Coronavirus Infection Prevention and Control guidance, aerosolisation rises with the use of high-speed surgical devices.[20] Ultrasonic devices work with the principle of high-frequency oscillation and hence theoretically a more potential aerosol generator. However, the magnitude of any such risks is unknown.[21]

8.3.C. Operating theatre environment

Usually, most of the traditional operating theatres have positive pressure ventilation relative to the surrounding air to prevent the flow of air from less sterile areas into a more sterile one. But this environment has a disadvantage in that it can spread the aerosols faster. So, there is a more chance of airborne viral transmission in such scenarios. Thus, it would be ideal to have an operation theatre with a negative pressure environment to reduce the dissemination of the virus beyond the operating theatre. A high frequency of filtered air exchanges can have added advantage in lowering viral load within an operating theatre.[22]

8.3.E. Open versus laparoscopic surgery

Although both open and laparoscopic surgery has the potential to generate aerosols, the overall risk seems to be lower with laparotomies as there is no requirement of creation of an artificial pneumoperitoneum. [23] Albeit the fact that the risk of aerosol spread may be lower during laparotomies, this theoretical risk must be balanced with the advantages we get from laparoscopic surgeries. Notably, less duration of hospital stay and earlier discharge can reduce nosocomial infections, thus decreasing the potential risk of SARS-CoV-2 infection and also will help in reducing the bed occupancy rate.[24-31] These advantages can provide much-needed capacity in terms of bed space and critical staff for health care institutions during this crucial time. [24-31]Brücher et al. found an equal risk of open and laparoscopic surgery if the gas/smoke was evacuated safely and with the use of water lock filters or if gasless laparoscopy was performed.[32]

8.4 Summary of current literature

Albeit theoretical risk, till date studies have rarely found SARS-CoV-2 in surgical smoke, and even if found, the infectivity of these viral particles are unknown. Although viral RNA may be detected in the blood, there is no evidence of transmission of COVID-19 through this route.[33] Similarly, although the viral DNA of blood-borne viral pathogens, such as hepatitis B and HIV, have been detected in surgical plume after the use of surgical energy, there is no evidence to indicate that their use increases the risk of disease transmission.[34,35] Moreover, Gynaecologists are well verged with surgery in patients with HIV and hepatitis B and C, without documented increased risk of transmission from the surgical plume or laparoscopic pneumoperitoneum. Further, there is no evidence from similar respiratory viruses, such as influenza, severe acute respiratory syndrome (SARS) or Middle East respiratory syndrome (MERS-CoV), about the virus to be transmitted through surgical plume or laparoscopic gas.[36] Thus the conclusion of the literature review is there is no compelling evidence to support the hypothesis that respiratory or blood-borne infectious viruses are transmitted through the surgical plume or aerosolised laparoscopic gas.

Thus, only with the theoretical background and without any evidence of transmission of SARS-COV-2 through the laparoscopic smoke plume or pneumoperitoneum, it's not justified to convert more number of cases to laparotomies which in turn can cost us the worst by consumption of precious resources (prolonged hospital stays and bed and manpower use), more significant number of surgical complications, and infectious exposure risks to the patient and the caregivers. Of course, despite the reassuring data, one should use adequate precautions to minimise any of the theoretic risks of transmission.

Hence the present scenario demands the role of a clinician in balancing the hypothetical risk of aerosol spread in low-risk patients to already established evidence of benefits of laparoscopic surgery.

8.5 Recommendations for laparoscopic surgery in suspected or confirmed COVID-19

Although there is no clear cut guideline, here we have summarised various national and international guidance (ISGE-2020, BSGE, 2020, ESGE, 2020, AAGL, 2020 etc.) for practical application during the COVID-19 situation.[2-

4,37,38] However, as the pandemic progresses and more date gathers, the guidance may be subjected to modification.

8.5.A. General considerations

- The Society of American Gastrointestinal and Endoscopic Surgeons (SAGE) and The European Society for Gynaecological Endoscopy (ESGE) have suggested postponing elective surgeries for benign conditions during the immediate phases of the pandemic.
- For conditions in which there is an existence of safe, nonsurgical alternative, the same should be explored to reduce the risk of horizontal transmission of SARS-CoV-2 virus.

8.5.B. Testing strategies

- A universal SARS-CoV-2 virology screening for patients planned for surgical treatment should be considered. But then this depends on the availability of the resources. Patients testing negative can proceed with the standard laparoscopic technique and routine surgical infection control procedures.
- Ideally, all preoperative patients should be tested if resources allow.
- Symptomatic patients must be tested.
- Imaging of the chest should be performed if clinically indicated, but this should not be used for screening.
- For those who screen or test negative, general anaesthesia and laparoscopic surgery can be considered with strict protocols of infection control.

- For those who screen or test positive, every attempt should be made to provide medical management and surgery should be delayed until the patient is recovered. Only emergency or life-saving surgery should be performed in such cases.
- Surgery should be undertaken with full PPE unless it can be safely postponed.
- Gynaecological operations carrying even a minimal risk of bowel involvement should be performed through laparotomies.

8.5.C. Anaesthetic considerations

- The patient should be advised to wear a respirator mask at all times.
- A full PPE should be worn by the anaesthetic staff.
- If possible intubation should be avoided, and every attempt should be made to utilise local or regional anaesthesia.
- If possible, the operating pressures should be minimised to reduce gas leaks whilst optimising ventilation. Positive airway pressure (Continuous positive airway pressure (CPAP) and bilevel positive airway pressure (BiPAP) should be avoided.
- To facilitate ventilatory needs trendelenburg position can be optimised, and this should be balanced between surgical and anaesthetic needs.

8.5.D. Operation theatre considerations

- All health workers should wear full PPE, irrespective of the test result of the patient.

- Preoperative chest X-ray or CT scan is of particular help for pulmonary assessment.
- Human resources in the operation theatre should be kept to a minimum to avoid unnecessary exposure.
- Ideally, negative pressure operation theatres should be utilised for patients who are positive or screen high risk, if available.
- Clear routes of entry and exit, donning, doffing, handling of specimens and sterilisation of instruments and theatres should be established, based on institutional infrastructure and resources. A straightforward Standard Operating Procedure (SOP) should be available for documenting these arrangements.

8.5.E. Strategies to reduce aerosol production

- The procedure should be performed by the most experienced surgeon available.
- The port taps should be closed before insertion.
- The incisions should of the appropriate size to prevent leakage during the procedure.
- The sound principles of energy should be utilised to optimise tissue effect.
- A CO_2 filter should be attached to one of the ports for smoke evacuation.
- The tap of all the ports should not be opened unnecessarily. Only those attached to a CO_2 filter or being used to deliver the gas can be opened.
- The frequency of introduction and removal of instruments through the ports should be minimised.

- Consider potential particle dispersion when choosing energy devices.
- Basic surgical principles should be employed i.e.
  - To minimise bleeding,
  - careful handling of tissue,
  - minimal use of energy at the lowest but effective settings and
  - use of atraumatic instruments.
- Caution should be maintained while using ultrasonic devices as the potential for aerosol generation may be higher. In this scenario avoidance of prolonged activation and the use of these devices in a low power setting can help minimise smoke production.
- Before removing the specimen bag from the abdomen, the latter should be deflated with a suction device through the port attached with a CO_2 filter.
- To minimise the use of cauterisation.
- Closed smoke evacuation systems should be used intraoperatively and at the end of the procedure, if available.

Wall suction connected to a central system is preferable to the use of mobile suctioning devices.

8.5.F. specimen retrieval and removal of the uterus at total laparoscopic hysterectomy

- It is advisable to use retrieval devices as it may minimise gas leaks.

- All colpocleiators (vaginal cuff delineators with air seal) should be checked preoperatively for gas leaks.
- Once the vault has been circumcised, all the gas should be removed by suction and/or closed system evacuators, before removing the specimen vaginally.

8.5.G. Port closure

- At present most of the guidelines support the practice of deflation prior to the removal of ports for the purpose of reducing aerosol spread.
- All ports should be removed only after the abdomen is deflated completely to reduce port site herniation.
- At the end of the procedure, the rectus sheath must be closed using a J needle at all the port-sites those are >10 mm size.
- As the commercial endoscopic port closure devices may allow for gas leaks, their use should be discouraged.

8.5.H. Postoperative strategies

- Every attempt should be made to employ same-day or early discharge where ever possible to avoid nosocomial infections.
- It's advisable to telephonically contact the postoperative patient to screen for postoperative symptoms after the surgery.

8.6 Hysteroscopy during COVID-19 pandemic

Although the theoretical risk of viral transmission through the generation of aerosol, is more significant during procedures such as laparoscopy or robotic surgery, this risk is minimal during hysteroscopy. This owes to the fact that hysteroscopy is not considered as an AGP and are not known to produce an aerosol. The use of electrosurgery in hysteroscopy is performed in a liquid environment. Bubbles that are generated with the help of thermal energy devices (monopolar, bipolar, or laser) are cooled down rapidly and partly absorbed by the surrounding liquid.[39] Cell fragments generated are contained within the uterine cavity.[40] Any gases that are volatile at ≤37°C and cell fragments are actively suctioned through the outflow channel, in a closed circuit, without an aerosol-generating effect, minimising any risk of viral dissemination. However, the actual risk is yet to be determined. Hence, Gynaecologists need to follow absolute careful consensus while conducting such procedures during the current pandemic.

8.7 Recommendations for hysteroscopic procedures during the COVID-19 pandemic

The following guidance represents a summary of statements issued by various international societies.[2-4, 37,38]

- The ongoing pandemic demands a postponement of all elective hysteroscopic procedures.

- Hysteroscopic procedures should be limited to emergency cases where delaying the procedure could result in deterioration of the patient's clinical condition.

- If possible, hysteroscopic procedures should be preferred to be performed in the office setting.

- A preoperative universal COVID-19 testing strategy should be adopted.

- ISGE recommends no anaesthesia or if indicated conscious sedation, local or regional anaesthesia for hysteroscopy.
- The entry of patient attendants should be restricted and a maximum of one adult attendant, under the age of 60 years, can be allowed with the patient when absolutely necessary.
- All healthcare members in close contact with the patient during the procedure should wear appropriate personal protective equipment (PPE).
- Only essential staff members should be allowed to stay, and the movement of staff members in and out of the procedure room should be restricted.
- During the procedure, multiple insertions and removals of the hysteroscope should be avoided from the uterine cavity.
- Training sessions should be organised by video transmission, and gathering of trainees should be avoided in the office or operating room.
- In patients with suspected or confirmed COVID-19 infection hysteroscopic procedure should be performed under strict protective environment and ideally in an operating room having negative pressure ventilation.
- An appropriate device should be selected such that it allows an effective and fast procedure.
- Nonsmoke generating devices such as hysteroscopic scissors, graspers, and tissue retrieval systems should be favoured to energy devices.

- As discussed earlier electrosurgery during hysteroscopy appears to generate less smoke than laparoscopy, although evidence to support this is yet to be found. In this regard, mechanical hysteroscopic morcellators have an upper hand advantage [41,42]
- The outflow tract should be connected with an active suction device. This is particularly important when using smoke-generating energy devices to facilitate the extraction of surgical smoke.
- When multiple cases are planned in the same room, sufficient time should be allowed in between procedures to perform thorough operating room decontamination.
- Early discharge of the patient should be considered.
- Standard endoscopic disinfection principle should be followed as these are quite effective.

8.8 Conclusion

Although there is a theoretic risk of airborne spread of SARS-CoV-2 from an abdominal source at the time of surgery, there is no evidence until now to prove this theory. Also, there is no current evidence in favour of the hypothesis that infection of health care personnel in the operation theatre occurs more commonly during laparoscopy than during laparotomy surgery. However, given the paucity of data, it is advised to take precautions in the operation theatres to combat the theoretical risk of airborne transmission and given the fact that viral particles can be aerosolised during intubation and extubation. For this reason, only emergency and cancer surgeries (where delaying the surgery may adversely affect the health condition of the patient) should be performed during this pandemic.

While performing laparoscopic hysterectomies, special care must be taken during colpotomy and subsequent uterine extraction to prevent and minimise unfiltered gas leakage. The abdomen should be emptied of gas using a suction device and filtered ports, as described above, prior to removal of the uterus. The decision to perform laparoscopy versus laparotomy should be taken on a case by case basis to minimise airborne droplet transmission.

The risk of aerosolisation is minimal during hysteroscopic surgeries compared to laparoscopy. However, due to the lack of experience and paucity of data during the current pandemic, it's prudent to take certain precautions as described.

8.9 References

1. Brindle M, Gawande A. Managing COVID-19 in surgical systems. Ann Surg. 2020; [Epub ahead of print].

2. 2.British Society for Gynaecological Endoscopy (BSGE). Joint RCOG BSGE Statement On Gynaecological Laparoscopic Procedures and Covid-19. 2020. https://www.bsge.org.uk/news/joint-rcog-bsge-statement-on-gynaecologicallaparoscopic-procedures-and-covid-19/.

3. 3.American Association of Gynecologic Laparoscopists (AAGL). COVID-19: Joint Statement on Minimally Invasive Gynecologic Surgery. 2020a. https://www.aagl.org/category/ covid-19/.

4. European Society for Gynaecological Endoscopy (ESGE). ESGE Recommendations on Gynaecological Laparoscopic Surgery during COVID-19 outbreak. Facts Views Vis Obgyn. 2020;12:5-6

5. Saridogan E, Grimbizis G. COVID-19 pandemic and gynaecological endoscopic surgery. Facts Views Vis Obgyn. 2020;12:1-3.

6. Alp E, Bijl D, Bleichrodt RP, Hansson B, Voss A. Surgical smoke and infection control. J Hosp Infect 2006';62(1):1–5.

7. Bree K, Barnhill S, Rundell W. The dangers of electrosurgical smoke to operating room personnel: a review. Workplace Health Saf 2017;65(11):517–26.

8. Capizzi PJ, Clay RP, Battey MJ. Microbiologic activity in laser resurfacing plume and debris. Lasers Surg Med 1998;23(3):172–4.

9. Johnson GK, Robinson WS. Human immunodeficiency virus-1 (HIV-1) in the vapors of surgical power instruments. J Med Virol 1991;33(1):47–50.

10. Kwak HD, Kim SH, Seo YS, Song KJ. Detecting hepatitis B virus in surgical smoke emitted during laparoscopic surgery. Occup Environ Med 2016;73 (12):857–63.

11. Setti L, Passarini F, De Gennaro G, et al. Airborne transmission route of COVID-19: why 2 meters/6 feet of inter-personal distance could not be enough. Int. J. Environ. Res. Public Health. 2020;17:E2932.

12. Van Doremalen N, Bushmaker T, Morris DH, et al. Aerosol and sur- face stability of SARS-CoV-2

as compared with SARS-CoV-1. N. Engl. J. Med. 2020;382:1564–1567.

13. Li CI, Pai JY, Chen CH. Characterisation of smoke generated during the use of surgical knife in laparotomy surgeries. J Air Waste Manag Assoc 2020;70 (3):324–32.

14. Liu Y, Song Y, Hu X, Yan L, Zhu X. Awareness of surgical smoke hazards and enhancement of surgical smoke prevention among the gynecologists. J Cancer 2019;10(12):2788

15. Meng L, Qiu H, Wan L et al. Intubation and Ventilation amid the COVID-19 Outbreak: Wuhan's Experience. Anesthesiology. 2020. Epub ahead of print.

16. Cho K, Hogan C, Lee M, Biswas P, Landman J, Champault G, Taffinder N, Ziol M, Riskalla H, Catheline JM (1997) Cells are present in the smoke created during laparoscopic surgery. Br J Surg 84(7):993–995

17. Knolmayer TJ, Asbun HJ, Shibata G, Bowyer MW (1977) An experimental model of cellular aerosolisation during laparoscopic surgery. Surg Laparosc Endosc 7(5):399–402

18. Ikramuddin S, Lucus J, Ellison EC, Schirmer WJ, Melvin WS (1998) Detection of aerosolised cells during carbon dioxide laparoscopy. J Gastrointest Surg 2(6):580–583

19. MallickR, Odejinmi F, Clark TJ.Covid 19 pandemic and gynaecological laparoscopic surgery: knowns and unknowns. Facts Views Vis Obgyn 2020;12(1):3

20. Department of Health and Social Care (DHSC), Public Health Wales (PHW), Public Health Agency

(PHA) Northern Ireland, Health Protection Scotland (HPS), Public Health England. COVID-19 guidance for infection prevention and control in healthcare settings. 2020.https:// assets.publishing.service.gov.uk/government/uploads/ system/uploads/attachment_data/file/874316/Infection_ prevention_and_control_guidance_for_pandemic_ coronavirus.pdf.

21. Zheng M, Boni L, Fingerhut A. Minimally invasive surgery and the novel coronavirus outbreak: lessons learned in China and Italy. Ann Surg. 2020. Epub ahead of print.

22. Wong J, Goh QY, Tan Z et al. Preparing for a COVID-19 pandemic: a review of operating room outbreak response measures in a large tertiary hospital in Singapore. Can J Anaesth. 2020. Epub ahead of print.

23. Li CI, Pai JY, Chen CH. Characterisation of smoke generated during the use of surgical knife in laparotomy surgeries. J Air Waste Manag Assoc 2020;70 (3):324–32.

24. Snyman LC, Makulana T, Makin JD. A randomised trial comparing laparoscopy with laparotomy in the management of women with ruptured ectopic pregnancy. S Afr Med J 2017;107(3):258–63.

25. Chapron C, Querleu D, Bruhat MA, et al. Surgical complications of diagnostic and operative gynaecological laparoscopy: a series of 29,966 cases. Hum Reprod 1998;13(4):867–72.

26. Mais V, Ajossa S, Guerriero S, Mascia M, Solla E, Melis GB. Laparoscopic versus abdominal myomectomy: a

prospective, randomised trial to evaluate benefits in early outcome. Am J Obstet Gynecol 1996;174(2):654–8.

27. Wen KC, Chen YJ, Sung PL, Wang PH. Comparing uterine fibroids treated by myomectomy through traditional laparotomy and 2 modified approaches: ultra-mini-laparotomy and laparoscopically assisted ultra-mini-laparotomy. Am J Obstet Gynecol 2010;202(2):144–e1.

28. Donnez O, Jadoul P, Squifflet J, Donnez J. A series of 3190 laparoscopic hysterectomies for benign disease from 1990 to 2006: evaluation of complications compared with vaginal and abdominal procedures. BJOG 2009;116(4):492–500.

29. Murphy AA, Nager CW, Wujek JJ, Kettel LM, Torp VA, Chin HG. Operative laparoscopy versus laparotomy for the management of ectopic pregnancy: a prospective trial. Fertil Steril 1992;57(6):1180–5.

30. Lundorff P, Thorburn J, Hahlin M, Källfelt B, Lindblom B. Laparoscopic surgery in ectopic pregnancy: a randomised trial versus laparotomy. Acta Obstet Gynecol Scand 1991;70(4-5):343–8.

31. Brill A, Ghosh K, Gunnarsson C, et al. The effects of laparoscopic cholecystectomy, hysterectomy, and appendectomy on nosocomial infection risks. Surg Endosc 2008;22(4):1112.

32. Brücher BL, Nigri G, Tinelli A, et al. COVID- 19: pandemic surgery guidance. 4open 2020;3:1.

33. Transfusion Transmitted Diseases Committee. Update: impact of 2019 novel Coronavirus and blood

safety. Available at: http://www.aabb.org/ advocacy/ regulatorygovernment/Documents/Impact-of-2019-NovelCoronavirus-on-Blood-Donation.pdf. Accessed March 28, 2020

34. Kwak HD, Kim SH, Seo YS, Song KJ. Detecting hepatitis B virus in surgical smoke emitted during laparoscopic surgery. Occup Environ Med. 2016;73:857–863.

35. Eubanks S, Newman L, Lucas G. Reduction of HIV transmission during laparoscopic procedures. Surg Laparosc Endosc. 1993;3:2–5.

36. Chang L, Yan Y, Wang L. Coronavirus disease 2019: Coronaviruses and blood safety. Transfus Med Rev. 2020 Feb 21. [Epub ahead of print].

37. SAGES - Society of American Gastrointestinal and Endoscopic Surgeons Recommendations Surgical Response to COVID 19. 2020 https://www.sages.org/recommendations-surgical-response-covid-19/

38. Thomas V, Maillard C, Barnard A, Snyman L, Chrysostomou A, Shimange-Matsose L et al. International Society for Gynecologic Endoscopy (ISGE) guidelines and recommendations on gynecological endoscopy during the evolutionary phases of the SARS-CoV-2 pandemic. European Journal of Obstetrics & Gynecology and Reproductive Biology. 2020;253:133-140.

39. Farrugia M. Electrosurgery on the uterus: an investigation of the local and systemic effects [dissertation]. London: University of London; 2009.

40. Farrugia M, Hussain SY, Perrett D. Particulate matter generated during monopolar and bipolar hysteroscopic human uterine tissue vaporisation. J Minim Invasive Gynecol. 2009;16:458–464.

41. The American College of Obstetricians and Gynaecologists (ACOG). Joint Statement on Elective Surgeries, 2020. Online March 16, http://www.acog.org/ news/news-releases/2020/03/joint-statement-on-elective-"www.acog.org/ news/news-releases/2020/03/joint-statement-on-elective-surgeries.

42. Donnez O, Jadoul P, Squifflet J, Donnez J. A series of 3190 laparoscopic hysterectomies for benign disease from 1990 to 2006: evaluation of complications compared with vaginal and abdominal procedures. BJOG 2009;116(4):492–500.

Chapter 9

Management of Gynaecological cancers during COVID-19 pandemic.

Dr. Soumya Ranjan Panda,

Assistant Professor, Department of Obstetrics and Gynecology, AIIMS, Mangalagiri, Andhra Pradesh

Abstract

In the current pandemic scenario, there is a higher demand for resuscitation and critical care services. So it would be prudent to reconsider the therapeutic options and indications. For the same reason, it's crucial to limit the infection rate in cancer patients. The current COVID-19 situation demands a patient prioritisation by considering the nature of the therapeutic strategy (curative versus palliative), their age, estimated life expectancy, and the timing of diagnosis. In the context of current COVID-19 pandemic, vaccination and screening programs can be delayed. For those patients who are found to have a low-grade cervical lesion on the screening test, the diagnostic evaluation may be postponed for 6-12 months. The first follow-up evaluation after treatment for high-grade lesions should not be delayed. A Multidisciplinary team should be involved in decision making of the modification of the standard of care to cope with the COVID-19 pandemic situation. Ideally, a decision of surgery should be made together with the patient. Counselling should be done about the risks of delaying surgery versus the risks of increased mortality and morbidity from developing COVID-19 perioperatively in hospital. The options of deferring surgery or nonsurgical treatments should be included and clearly documented during the informed consent process.

9.1 Background

In spite of infliction of measures like quarantine, nationwide lockdown, social distancing, and hygiene education, the COVID-19 spread, unfortunately, continues with different patterns of occurrence in a different part of the world.[1] Susceptibility and disease severity seems higher in patients who have other comorbidities. Cancerous patients are such a group, who appear to be more susceptible to COVID-19. The risk is even more severe for those who have a history of recent surgery or chemotherapy. A report from China, published in mid-February 2020, found a 3.5 times higher risk in terms of mechanical ventilation need, intensive care admission, or death in patients with a history of cancer.[2] CovidSurg project, is an ongoing international multi-centre study, analysing data from COVID-19 operated patients. A high overall mortality rate (24%) and pulmonary complication rate (51%) has been found. The most common cause of mortality was pulmonary complications, and a 19% mortality risk was found to be associated with elective surgeries. Hence the data is in favour of postponing elective surgeries during the ongoing pandemic.[3]

In the current pandemic scenario, there is a higher demand for resuscitation and critical care services. So it would be prudent to reconsider the therapeutic options and indications. For the same reason, it's crucial to limit the infection rate in cancer patients. Two important priorities should be considered to reduce the risk of infections A) to avoid high-risk procedures such as surgery and chemotherapy as far as possible and B) to reduce the patient's contact with healthcare workers and with places of care. Thus, to achieve the above priorities among gynecologic cancer patients, all the alternative options to surgery must be explored while bearing in mind that the main objective for these patients remains therapeutic management. In particular, it would be ideal to analyse the risk-benefit ratio for surgical procedures on a case-by-case basis.

9.2 General considerations

Conventionally the therapeutic options of oncologic patients are based on two strategies:

1) Curative treatment is intended for localised diseases, or some advanced/metastatic cancers and depending upon the sensitivity and the disease course can be of medical, surgical or radiotherapeutic treatment

2) Palliative (non-curative) treatment option is adopted for diseases too advanced to be curable.

The current COVID-19 situation demands a patient prioritisation by considering the kind of the therapeutic option (curative or palliative), their age, estimated life expectancy, and the timing of diagnosis.

Given the high percentage of asymptomatic patients and the high infectivity of SARS-COV-2, all pathologic samples should be considered as potentially infected. Recently it was reported that fixation in formalin could inactivate the SARS-COV-2 virus. Although there is an associated risk of toxicity related to formalin exposure, this appears to be less serious than that related to the exposure of fresh, non-fixed tissue potentially carrying the virus.

9.3 Cervical cancer

In the context of a current pandemic, the option like radiotherapy or concomitant chemoradiation should be favoured as first-line treatment whenever possible in place of surgery. Especially, the need for lymph node dissection should be reviewed on a case-by-case basis upon considering the site, imaging reports and the disease stage. Hysterectomy after concomitant chemoradiation should only be indicated for any post-therapeutic tumour residue.

Albeit the fact that surgery is the preferred treatment modality in patients with early-stage cervical cancer, it can be avoided in two particular classes of patients. First, in the elderly (aged >70 years) patients affected by early-stage cervical cancer, primary radiotherapy can be adopted as an alternative to surgery. Second, for those early-stage cervical cancers with tumours larger than 2 cm and a sign of the encroachment of stromal ring (detected at preoperative workup), definitive radiotherapy (with or without chemotherapy)should be offered as an alternative therapeutic option. [4]

Various organisations have classified the clinical conditions to prioritise the treatment during this pandemic.

9.3.A Management of Vaccination and Screening Programs During and After the COVID-19 Pandemic. [5-14]

In the context of current COVID-19 pandemic, vaccination and screening programs can be delayed. But this decision should be based on cervical cancer epidemiology, the transmission pattern of SARS-COV-2, locally adopted containment measures, and health and immunisation system resources. Provision of such facilities can be suspended till authorities in charge of COVID-19 control feel that mobility of the target population and healthcare givers must be restricted to minimise SARS-CoV-2 transmission. [14,15]

The backlog cases resulting due to the above measures should be handled with careful planning so as to affect the drops minimally in mid- and long-term population coverage. Measures should be adopted to complete the vaccination schedule for those who have already started on HPV vaccination. In these cases, an interval of less than 12–15 months from the first dose should be maintained.[9]

9.3 B Management of Screen-Positive Women

After reviewing the recent interim guidelines related to COVID-19, following points can be summarised and is applicable for the current pandemic situation.[5-14]

For those patients who are found to have low-grade cervical cancer ("normal cervical cytology with a positive high-risk HPV test," "low grade squamous intraepithelial lesion (LSIL)," or "atypical squamous cells of undetermined significance (ASC-US) with a positive high-risk HPV test") on a screening test, diagnostic evaluation (colposcopy) may be postponed for 6-12 months. For example, a colposcopy can be deferred for 6-12 months for lesions such as if clinical symptoms are absent.

On the other hand, lesions such as "squamous cell carcinoma," "atypical glandular cells- favour neoplasia (AGC-FN)," "endocervical adenocarcinoma in situ," or "adenocarcinoma" are considered to have the highest risk. Hence these should be evaluated as soon as possible preferably within 4weeks from the results.

Similarly, a time period of one to three month can be allowed to evaluate lesions such as "high grade squamous intraepithelial lesion (HSIL)," "atypical squamous cells that cannot exclude HSIL (ASC-H)," or "atypical glandular cells not otherwise specified (AGS-NOS)" and colposcopy can be deferred for 1 to 3months from the time of availability of results.

9.3.C *Management of Preinvasive and Invasive Lesions of the Lower Genital Tract*

Patients with a confirmed diagnosis of invasive cancer as on histopathology report of cervical, vaginal, or vulval biopsy should be contacted within two weeks. Similarly, patients with symptoms suspicious for lower genital tract cancers should also undergo evaluation within two weeks.

A histopathological diagnosis of high-grade cervical (CIN2–3), vaginal (VAIN2–3), or vulvar (VIN2-3 or differentiated VIN) intraepithelial lesion should prompt clinicians for its surgical treatment within three months from diagnosis. [16] A conservative approach can be offered to patients with CIN2,

VAIN2, or VIN2 provided the first scheduled appointment can be arranged at 6th month. However, physical appointments can be postponed up to 12 months for a histopathological diagnosis of a low-grade intraepithelial lesion from a cervical, vaginal, or vulvar biopsy/excision.[16]

The first follow-up evaluation after treatment for high-grade lesions should not be delayed. Essentially, the first follow-up evaluation at the sixth month from treatment should include high-risk HPV test or high-risk HPV test with cervical cytology in the case of CIN2-3 or VAIN2-3. A vulvoscopy should be done in the case of VIN2-3 or differentiated VIN.

Resumption of elective diagnostic and surgical procedures for preinvasive, invasive or other lower genital tract pathologies should be done based on several aspects of the COVID-19 pandemic like sustained reduction rate of new COVID-19 cases, adequate availability of personal protective equipment and prompt availability of COVID-19 testing program for staff and patient safety etc.[17]

9.4 Ovarian cancer

9.4.A. Primary surgical treatment of ovarian cancer

A combined surgical and chemotherapeutical approach remains the mainstay of treatment for patients with ovarian cancer. The treatment modality of ovarian cancer depends upon the stage of presentation and patient characteristics. Even during the period of COVID-19 pandemic, surgery should be the form of management for early stages of ovarian cancer. In these cases, surgery with or without chemotherapy facilitate tumour debulking, staging and causes a high probability of long-term cure.[18]

The option of lymphadenectomy should be tailored based on patient and disease characteristics, especially for early-stage ovarian cancer. Where ever possible, it should be avoided. As far as histopathologic tumour type is concerned, lymphadenectomy should be avoided in mucinous tumours but can be performed in other histological types (e.g., serous histology) at high risk of nodal spread.[19] There is no data to support the beneficial effects of full lymphadenectomy in these patients, especially if adjuvant chemotherapy is planned.[19]

In advanced stages of ovarian cancer (stage IIIB–IV) surgery followed adjuvant chemotherapy remains as the standard of care.[18] However, recently there is growing evidence in favour of the alternative option of neoadjuvant chemotherapy followed by interval debulking surgery for these advanced stages of ovarian cancer. Neoadjuvant chemotherapy followed by interval debulking surgery appears to reduce morbidity related to surgeries (since there is a reduction of complex nature of surgery) and has been found to have a similar long-term outcome compared to the primary cytoreductive surgery. There are two randomised controlled trials (EORTC5597 and the CHORUS study) those reported the non-inferiority and less invasiveness of neoadjuvant chemotherapy followed by interval debulking surgery compared to primary cytoreductive surgery in patients affected by the advanced disease.[20] Moreover, there is a matter of concern related to primary debulking surgery that less number of patients achieve complete (no residual disease) and optimal (residual disease<1 cm) cytoreduction. [21] Another ongoing study (TRUST) will clarify the role of neoadjuvant chemotherapy in advanced-stage ovarian cancer.[22] Based on the above the literature, the use of primary cytoreductive surgery should be avoided in the context of COVID-19 pandemic for whom the extensive cytoreductive procedure is anticipated. Also, the neoadjuvant chemotherapy reduces treatment-related morbidity and may possibly facilitate the execution of surgery after a certain time period. Histological assessment is essential before starting of chemotherapy which can be achieved by laparoscopic examination or radiological-guided biopsy. Hence a decision to have primary cytoreductive surgery in advanced staged ovarian cancer with a high burden of disease should be carefully discussed and should be reserved in a selected group of patients.

9.4.B Surgical treatment of recurrent ovarian cancer

Secondary cytoreductive surgery in recurrent ovarian cancer is an important issue to be considered. Generally, those patients with only a few metastatic diseases and long-term progression-free survival are ideal candidates for Secondary cytoreductive surgery. Accumulating literature has shown that secondary and tertiary cytoreductive surgery might improve outcomes of ovarian cancer patients if complete cytoreduction can be achieved.[23-25] The randomised phase III trial AGO DESKTOP OVAR III is an ongoing study evaluating the role of secondary cytoreduction followed by chemotherapy compared to chemotherapy alone bears the hope to through some clarity on the role of surgery in patients with recurrent ovarian cancer.[26] However, the only randomised trial (GOG 213) evaluating the role of secondary surgery in patients with recurrent ovarian cancers failed to demonstrate any positive effect of surgery in these patients. [27] Additionally, patient-reported quality of life was significantly low after surgery although there was no significant difference between the two groups after recovery. [27] Hence, based on the supporting evidence in favour of chemotherapy only as of the therapeutic option for recurrent ovarian cancer patients, the secondary surgery should be reserved only for the highly selected patients especially during the COVID-19 outbreak.

9.4.C Palliative surgery for ovarian cancer

Palliative care is adopted to relieve the symptoms, and pain related to end-stage ovarian cancer. Hence it is essential for maintaining a quality of life and should not be avoided if clinical judgement favours the necessity. The indications for palliative surgery include Bowel obstruction, persistent pelvic pain, fistula formation, tumour necrosis, pelvic sepsis, and chronic haemorrhage. Bowel obstruction is the primary indication for palliative surgery in patients with end-stage ovarian cancer. instead of bowel resection and bypass, ostomies should be performed to achieve relief of bowel obstructions. [28] An attempt with medical management should be adopted before advising surgery. During the current pandemic, palliative chemotherapy and/or stereotactic body radiotherapy should be considered in preference to surgeries.

9.5 Endometrial cancer

Early-stage cancers

Surgical treatment is the preferred option for early-stage endometrial cancer. However, for low-risk endometrial cancers (FIGO Ia stage on MRI and grade 1–2 endometrioid cancer on endometrial biopsy) surgery can be delayed for 1–2 months if one does not find any discrepancy on the initial assessments, particularly if the patient is elderly and / or with comorbidities.[4] Hence in the context of COVID-19 pandemic, the following options can be considered. For low-risk Grade 1 disease Hormonal therapy[29]51 or delayed surgery for 1–2 months (grade 1–2 stage 1A, MRI confirmed) can be adopted.[4] On the other hand, for high-risk grade 2/3 disease hysterectomy and bilateral salpingo-oophorectomy with or without sentinel lymph node assessment depending upon the availability. In patients who are at high anaesthetic risk, radiotherapy instead of surgery can be considered.[30,31]

Advanced stage cancers

For advanced endometrial cancers (stages III and IV), first-line medical treatment should be administered.[4] In early-stage disease, delaying methods such as using the levonorgestrel-releasing intrauterine system or oral progesterone may be used. [32] In advanced stage or recurrent disease, Megestrol/megestrol alternating with tamoxifen (endometrioid histology/estrogen, progesterone receptor-positive); oral everolimus/letrozole or Neoadjuvant chemotherapy may be used. [4,32,33]

For suspected endometrial cancer

For patients presenting with postmenopausal bleeding and endometrial thickening on ultrasound, endometrial sampling with a pipelle should be done in consultation. A diagnostic hysteroscopy in the consultation should be avoided unless performed at the same visit (to limit the number of patient visits). In the event of an equivocal diagnostic assessment, the appointment of the diagnostic hysteroscopy and curettage should be based on the degree of suspicion of endometrial cancer and the constraints of access to the operating room. For example, If the risk of cancer appears to be low and the patient is elderly, the procedure under general anaesthesia can be delayed until after the confinement period for COVID-19.[4]

9.6 Gestational trophoblastic neoplasia

Although trophoblastic tumours have a high metastatic potential, these are considered one of the most curable tumour. So any delay in treating these patients should not be entertained even during this pandemic. Patients with low-risk trophoblastic tumours treatment can be done with methotrexate while those with high-risk tumours should be treated with multi-drug regimens without delay (chemotherapy with curative intent).[34,35] Conventional curettage should be offered as it bears both a diagnostic as well as a therapeutic value (~40% of patients subsequently do not require chemotherapy). [36,37] Hysterectomy may be offered, for those with family completed.[35,37] For patients with high-risk disease, inpatient management with multi-drug regimens should be offered.

9.7 Conclusion

A Multidisciplinary team should be involved in decision making of the modification of the standard of care to cope with the COVID-19 pandemic situation. Ideally, a decision of surgery should be made together with the patient. Counselling should be done about the risks of delaying surgery versus the risks of increased mortality and morbidity from developing COVID-19 perioperatively in hospital. In addition to the usual consent form, a supplementary consent form documenting the increased rate of mortality and morbidity related to COVID-19 disease around the time of cancer treatment should be used. The possibility of worsening survival if treatment is delayed should be outlined to patients. The options of deferring surgery or nonsurgical treatments should also be included and clearly documented during the informed consent process.

9.8 Reference

1. Johns Hopkins University. COVID-19 dashboard by the centre for systems science and engineering at Johns Hopkins University [Internet]. Baltimore, MD: Johns Hopkins University; c2020 [cited 2020 Apr 20]. Available from: https://coronavirus.jhu.edu/map.html.

2. Liang W, Guan W, Chen R, et al. Cancer patients in SARSCoV-2 infection: a nationwide analysis in China. Lancet Oncol 2020;21:335–7.

3. Nepogodiev D, Glasbey JC, Li E, et al. Mortality and pulmonary complications in patients undergoing surgery with perioperative SARS-CoV-2 infection: an international cohort study. Lancet 2020. doi:10.1016/S0140-6736(20)31182-X. [Epub ahead of print: 29 May 2020].

4. Akladios C, Azais H, Ballester M, Bendifallah S, Bolze P, Bourdel N et al. Recommendations for the surgical management of gynecological cancers during the COVID-19 pandemic - FRANCOGYN group for the CNGOF. Journal of Gynecology Obstetrics and Human Reproduction. 2020;49(6):101729.

5. Sundar S, Wood N, Ghaem-Maghami S, et al. BGCS RCOG framework for care of patients with gynaecological cancer during the COVID-19 pandemic, 2020. Available: https://www.bgcs.org.uk/wpcontent/uploads/2020/05/BGCS-guidance-v-3-final_-1.pdf

6. Sebastianelli A, Plante M, Langlais E, et al. GOC position statement for the COVID-19 pandemic situation: treatment and management for women with gynecologic cancer, 2020. Available: http:// g-o-c.org/wp-content/uploads/2020/04/20GOC_COVID-19_PositionStatement_FINAL_Apr7.pdf [Accessed 24 Apr 2020].

7. Lee S-J, Kim T, Kim M, et al. Recommendations for gynecologic cancer care during the COVID-19 pandemic. J Gynecol Oncol 2020;31.

8. Ramirez PT, Chiva L, Eriksson AGZ, et al. COVID-19 global pandemic: options for management of gynecologic cancers. Int J Gynecol Cancer 2020;30:561–3.

9. British Society for Colposcopy and Cervical Pathology. NHS cervical screening programme: Colposcopy initial guidance during the coronavirus (Covid-19) pandemic, 2020. Available: https://www.bsccp.org.uk/assets/file/uploads/resources/0_PHE_%28England%29_Guidance_for_Colposcopy_Service_Providers_V1_0.pdf [Accessed 3 May 2020].

10. British Society for Colposcopy and Cervical Pathology. Colposcopy guidance during COVID 19 pandemic, 2020. Available: https://www. bsccp.org.uk/assets/

file/uploads/resources/Colposcopy_guidance__COVID_19_pandemic.V3.pdf [Accessed 27 May 2020].

11. Ciavattini A, Delli Carpini G, Giannella L, et al. Expert consensus from the Italian Society for Colposcopy and Cervico-Vaginal Pathology (SICPCV) for colposcopy and outpatient surgery of the lower genital tract during the COVID-19 pandemic. Int J Gynaecol Obstet 2020;149:269–72.

12. European Society for Medical Oncology. ESMO management and treatment adapted recommendations in the COVID-19 era: cervical cancer, 2020. Available: https://www.esmo.org/guidelines/cancer-patient-management-during-the-covid-19-pandemic/gynaecological-malignancies-cervical-cancer-in-the-covid-19-era [Accessed 27 May 2020].

13. Cibula D, Gultekin M, McCormack M, et al. Management of cervical cancer during the COVID-19 pandemic, 2020. Available: https://eacademy.esgo.org/esgo/2020/covid-19/298855/david.cibula.murat.gultekin.mary.mccormack.domenica.lorusso.pedro.ramirez.html?f=listing=3*browseby=8*sortby=2*media=1*label=19832*featured=16722 [Accessed 25 May 2020].

14. Ciavattini A, Delli Carpini G, Giannella L, et al. European Federation for Colposcopy (EFC) and European Society of Gynaecological Oncology (ESGO) joint considerations about human papillomavirus (HPV) vaccination, screening programs, colposcopy, and surgery during and after the COVID-19 pandemic.

Int J Gynecol Cancer 2020. doi:10.1136/ijgc-2020-001617. [Epub ahead of print: 02 Jun 2020].

15. Recommendations for gynecologic cancer care during the COVID-19 pandemic. Journal of Gynecologic Oncology. 2020;31(4).

16. Castle PE, Adcock R, Cuzick J, et al. Relationships of p16 immunohistochemistry and other biomarkers with diagnoses of cervical abnormalities: implications for last terminology. Arch Pathol Lab Med 2019. doi:10.5858/arpa.2019-0241-OA

17. American College of Surgeons. Joint statement: roadmap for resuming elective surgery after COVID-19 pandemic. Available: https://www.facs.org/covid-19/clinical-guidance/roadmap-electivesurgery [Accessed 10 May 2020].

18. Peres LC, Sinha S, Townsend MK, Fridley BL, Karlan BY, Lutgendorf SK, et al. Predictors of survival trajectories among women with epithelial ovarian cancer. Gynecol Oncol 2020;156:459-66. PUBMED | CROSSREF

19. Bogani G, Tagliabue E, Ditto A, Signorelli M, Martinelli F, Casarin J, et al. Assessing the risk of pelvic and para-aortic nodal involvement in apparent early-stage ovarian cancer: a predictors- and nomogram-based analyses. Gynecol Oncol 2017;147:61-5. PUBMED | CROSSREF

20. Vergote I, Coens C, Nankivell M, Kristensen GB, Parmar MK, Ehlen T, et al. Neoadjuvant chemotherapy versus debulking surgery in advanced tubo-ovarian

cancers: pooled analysis of individual patient data from the EORTC 55971 and CHORUS trials. Lancet Oncol 2018;19:1680-7. PUBMED | CROSSREF

21. Bogani G, Leone Roberti Maggiore U, Paolini B, Diito A, Martinelli F, Lorusso D, et al. The detrimental effect of adopting interval debulking surgery in advanced stage low-grade serous ovarian cancer. J Gynecol Oncol 2019;30:e4. PUBMED | CROSSREF

22. Reuss A, du Bois A, Harter P, Fotopoulou C, Sehouli J, Aletti G, et al. TRUST: Trial of Radical Upfront Surgical Therapy in advanced ovarian cancer (ENGOT ov33/AGO-OVAR OP7). Int J Gynecol Cancer 2019;29:1327-31. PUBMED | CROSSREF

23. Bogani G, Rossetti D, Ditto A, Martinelli F, Chiappa V, Mosca L, et al. Artificial intelligence weights the importance of factors predicting complete cytoreduction at secondary cytoreductive surgery for recurrent ovarian cancer. J Gynecol Oncol 2018;29:e66. PUBMED | CROSSREF

24. Harter P, Hahmann M, Lueck HJ, Poelcher M, Wimberger P, Ortmann O, et al. Surgery for recurrent ovarian cancer: role of peritoneal carcinomatosis: exploratory analysis of the DESKTOP I Trial about risk factors, surgical implications, and prognostic value of peritoneal carcinomatosis. Ann Surg Oncol 2009;16:1324-30. PUBMED | CROSSREF

25. Harter P, Sehouli J, Reuss A, Hasenburg A, Scambia G, Cibula D, et al. Prospective validation study of a

predictive score for operability of recurrent ovarian cancer: the Multicenter Intergroup Study DESKTOP II. A project of the AGO Kommission OVAR, AGO Study Group, NOGGO, AGO-Austria, and MITO. Int J Gynecol Cancer 2011;21:289-95. PUBMED | CROSSREF

26. Bogani G, Tagliabue E, Signorelli M, Ditto A, Martinelli F, Chiappa V, et al. A score system for complete cytoreduction in selected recurrent ovarian cancer patients undergoing secondary cytoreductive surgery: predictors- and nomogram-based analyses. J Gynecol Oncol 2018;29:e40. PUBMED | CROSSREF

27. Coleman RL, Spirtos NM, Enserro D, Herzog TJ, Sabbatini P, Armstrong DK, et al. Secondary surgical cytoreduction for recurrent ovarian cancer. N Engl J Med 2019;381:1929-39. PUBMED | CROSSREF

28. Hope JM, Pothuri B. The role of palliative surgery in gynecologic cancer cases. Oncologist 2013;18:73-9. PUBMED | CROSSREF

29. Ramirez PT, Chiva L, Eriksson AGZ, et al. COVID-19 global pandemic: options for management of gynecologic cancers. Int J Gynecol Cancer 2020;30:561–3.

30. Lee S-J, Kim T, Kim M, et al. Recommendations for gynecologic cancer care during the COVID-19 pandemic. J Gynecol Oncol 2020;31.

31. Royal College of Radiologists. Royal College of Radiologists radiotherapy dose fractionation, Third edition: Cervix cancer, 2019. Available: https://www.

rcr.ac.uk/system/files/publication/field_ publication_ files/bfco193_radiotherapy_dose_fractionation_ thirdedition-gynaecological-cancers_0.pdf [Accessed 3 May 2020].

32. Pothuri B, Alvarez Secord A, Armstrong DK, et al. Anti-cancer therapy and clinical trial considerations for gynecologic oncology patients during the COVID-19 pandemic crisis. Gynecol Oncol 2020. doi:10.1016/j. ygyno.2020.04.694. [Epub ahead of print: 23 Apr 2020].

33. COVID-19: global consequences for oncology. Lancet Oncol 2020;21:467.

34. Akladios C, Azais H, Ballester M, et al. Recommendations for the surgical management of gynecological cancers during the COVID-19 pandemic - FRANCOGYN group for the CNGOF. J Gynecol Obstet Hum Reprod 2020;49.

35. Sebastianelli A, Plante M, Langlais E, et al. GOC position statement for the COVID-19 pandemic situation: treatment and management for women with gynecologic cancer, 2020. Available: http:// g-o-c.org/ wp-content/uploads/2020/04/20GOC_COVID-19_ PositionStatement_FINAL_Apr7.pdf [Accessed 24 Apr 2020]

36. Society of Gynecologic Oncology. Gynecologic oncology considerations during the COVID-19 pandemic, 2020. Available: https://www.sgo.org/clinical-practice/ management/covid-19- resources-for-health-care-

practitioners/gyn-onc-considerationsduring-covid-19/ [Accessed 24 Apr 2020].

37. Dowdy S, Fader AN. Surgical considerations for gynecologic oncologists during the COVID-19 pandemic, 2020. Available: https://www.sgo.org/wp-content/uploads/2020/03/Surgical_ Considerations_ Communique.v14.pdf [Accessed 25 Apr 2020].

Chapter 10

COVID-19 pandemic and impact on Maternal psychological health

1. Dr. Jaiganesh Selvapandiyan

Assistant Professor, Department of Psychiatry, AIIMS, Mangalagiri, Andhra Pradesh

2. Dr. Soumya Ranjan Panda,

Assistant Professor, Department of Obstetrics and Gynecology, AIIMS, Mangalagiri, Andhra Pradesh

Abstract

Self-isolation, quarantine and lockdowns are some of the inflicted measures taken to combat the disease spread. Thus for a certain group of the population, it's quite obvious to experience mental health problems to deal with such a calamity and the sudden social changes related to it. Although pregnancy is a special stage in a woman's life, the journey is not smooth always. While some women may have to encounter some negative thoughts and emotions during pregnancy leading to anxiety and depression, others may have to deal with some form of stress. Some individuals may get involved in harmful acts such as alcohol consumption or substance abuse to overcome the crisis stage, thus aggravating existing psychological problems. This may end up in an increased incidence of domestic violence, an increase in suicide rates, especially among low -income families and immigrant communities. Women should be assessed for any pre-existing mental health conditions or substance use disorders, and these should be addressed through mental health services early in pregnancy. Women should be educated (preferably in the local language)about the latest facts of COVID-19 affecting pregnant women and infants, as well as about the preventive and safety measures that should be adopted. To care for the psychological health of pregnant women is as important as to deal with the pandemic. Therefore it is important to develop appropriate strategies to screen for important psychological issues especially stress, depression, domestic violence etc. and to address other issues related to perinatal mental health disorders during the current pandemic, without delay.

10.1 Background

With the pandemic of Coronavirus disease -19 (COVID -19) creating havoc, every possible way is being adopted by the medical communities and various governments around the world to halt the spread. Self-isolation, quarantine and lockdowns are some of the inflicted measures taken to combat the disease spread. Thus for a certain group of the population, it's quite obvious to experience mental health problems to deal with such a calamity and the sudden social changes related to it. Recently few studies have reported a higher prevalence of mental health problems among women compared to men. [1] As such, pregnant women and new mothers could certainly be more vulnerable. Although pregnancy is a special stage in a woman's life, the journey is not smooth always. While some women may have to encounter some negative thoughts and emotions during pregnancy leading to anxiety and depression, others may have to deal with some form of stress. Maternal mental health problems can be associated with short-term and long-term risks for the affected mother as well as for their children in terms of physical, cognitive and psychological development. Moreover, certain conditions like extreme stress, emergency situations and natural disasters can inflate the risks of perinatal mental health morbidity. Therefore, it is obvious that pregnant women are vulnerable to mental ill-health during the COVID-19 pandemic.

10.2 The Burden of mental health during the pandemic

Strict public health measures directed towards combating the spread of disease, although quite essential, but may lead to negative psychological effects resulting in stress, anger and confusion.[2] In this context concerns regarding the wellbeing of the unborn child, the prolonged pandemic chaos and the related economic consequences etc. are likely to further escalate psychological burden and worsen the mental wellbeing of pregnant women and new mothers. Less studied facts related to the effects of COVID-19 on pregnancy and the foetus is likely to add further to psychological stress. Some individuals may get involved in harmful acts such as alcohol consumption or substance abuse to overcome the crisis stage, thus aggravating existing psychological problems. This may also result in an increase in domestic violence, an increase in suicide rates, especially among low-income families and immigrant communities.

Specifically in India, there is an acute shortage of health care personnel in the rural areas. The strength of health staff in these areas is much below the bench mark advocated by WHO that is, 22.8 health workers per 10 000 populations.[3] Again, the current doctor population ratio in India (1:1445) is far below the WHO's prescribed norm (1:1000). Moreover, there is only one-fourth of the doctors in rural areas of India as compared to urban areas.[4,5] Another factor that shortage of personal protective equipments forces the rural health care personnel to perform their duties without proper precautionary measures. These factors contribute to raise the anxiety level amongst the pregnant women and lactating mothers on fear of being infected.[6]

During the perinatal period, there is a good chance of getting affected by depression and anxiety. The changing hormonal lieu could one of the contributing factor. It has been found that approximately one in seven women during the perinatal period could be affected by depression and anxiety.[7] Postpartum Depression (PPD) has been found in as many as 22% of Indian mothers. This is also known as 'baby blues', that disturbs a woman's ability to take care of her baby and herself.[8,9]

In this critical situation, every community in the world is going through a tough struggle and are trying their best to combat an unfamiliar disease. Equally important, even during such a calamity, is the need to scrutinise for any new threats to pregnant women and infants.[10] However, mental health needs are currently overshadowed by other, more pressing issues in healthcare.

10.3 Guidance for the care of maternal psychological health.[11]

1) Women-centred care should be Provided during telehealth consultations ensuring that the woman's priorities are addressed and supporting them in opting altered prenatal care services.

2) Women should be educated (preferably in the local language)about the latest facts of COVID-19 affecting pregnant women and infants, as well as about the preventive and safety measures that should be adopted.

3) Women should be assessed for any pre-existing mental health conditions or substance use disorders, and these should be addressed through mental health services early in pregnancy. They also should be screened for domestic and intimate partner violence, and referrals should be provided to psychological health and social services, as well as other concerned organisations, which can provide safety planning, cognitive behavioural therapy, and other ongoing support.

4) It should be born in mind that communities affected by systemic racism, housing instability, low socioeconomic status, poor access to health care etc. are increasingly sensitive to get affected by COVID-19. These group of the population may be unable to consistently practice infection control measures and social distancing and are at increased risk for poor mental health outcomes and inadequate social support.

5) It should be acknowledged that labor and birth in a pandemic are not according to the mother's expectations or planning and that feelings of anxiety, sadness, grief, fear, or loss are normal.

6) Infant- mother bond should be maintained, and it should be avoided to separate mothers and infants unless required by clinical condition.

7) Skin-to-skin care and breastfeeding should be promoted as long as it's safely possible. Infants who are separated from mothers should be observed for excessive stress and ensuring that human touch is provided to these infants.

8) It's better to reevaluate psychological symptoms (stress, depression, anxiety), support systems, and safety upon discharge to assess for community care needs.

9) Women should be made to access to virtual and community mental health resources while maintaining social distancing. Collaborative networks should be created with the community-based organisations to enhance coordination and optimisation of care. For pregnant and postpartum women who are working as health care or other frontline workers, mental health resources and support should be advocated.

10.4 Conclusion

The psychological health of pregnant women is an important aspect to care for during the current pandemic. Thus, government agencies should be actively involved in developing appropriate strategies to screen for important psychological issues especially stress, depression, domestic violence etc. and to address other issues related to perinatal mental health disorders during the current pandemic, without delay. Internet-based screening tools, virtual online consultations/counselling and web-based psychological support and therapeutic interventions may have an important role in this regard.

10.5 References

1. 1.Liu N, Zhang F, Wei C, Jia Y, Shang Z, Sun L, et al. Prevalence and predictors of PTSS during COVID -19 outbreak in China hardest-hit areas: Gender differences matter. Psychiatry Res. 2020;287:112921.

2. Brooks SK, Webster RK, Smith LE, et al., The psychological impact of quarantine and how to reduce it: rapid review of the evidence. Lancet . 2020 ,395(10227):912 -920.

3. 3.Shekhar V. Covid-19 and demand for maternal health services. *The Indian Express.* 2020. https://indianexpress.com/article/opinion/covid-19-and-demand-for-maternal-health-services-6410678/.

4. 4.Press Trust of India. India's doctor-patient ratio still behind WHO-prescribed 1:1,000: Govt. *Business Standard.* 2019. https://www.business-standard.com/article/pti-stories/doctor-patient-ratio-in-india-less-than-who-prescribed-norm-of-1-1000-govt-119111901421_1.html.

5. 5.Munjal A. We don't have enough doctors in rural India. That's why we need telemedicine. *BW Disrupt.* 2017. http://bwdisrupt.businessworld.in/article/We-Don-t-Have-Enough-Doctors-in-Rural-India-That-s-Why-We-Need-Telemedicine-/14-06-2017-120121/

6. 2Bisht R, Sarma J, Saharia R. COVID-19 lockdown: guidelines are not enough to ensure pregnant women receive care. *The Wire.* 2020; https://thewire.in/women/covid-19-lockdown-pregnant-women-childbirth.

7. Davenport MH, Meyer S, Meah VL, Strynadka MC, Khurana R. Moms are not ok: COVID-19 and maternal mental health. *Frontiers in Global Women's Health.* 2020; **1**: 1. https://doi.org/10.3389/fgwh.2020.00001.

8. Upadhyay RP, Chowdhury R, Salehi A, Sarkar K, Singh SK, Sinha B, Pawar A, Rajalakshmi AK, Kumar A. Postpartum depression in India: a systematic review and meta-analysis. *Bull World Health Organ.* 2017; **95**(10): 706– 717B. https://doi.org/10.2471/BLT.17.192237.

9. Medha. 22% of new mothers in India suffer from postpartum depression: WHO. *Medical Dialogues.* 2018. https://speciality.medicaldialogues.in/22-of-new-mothers-in-india-suffer-from-postpartum-depression-who

10. Frey MT, Meaney -Delman D, Bowen V, et al., Surveillance for Emerging Threats to Pregnant Women and Infants. J Womens Health (Larchmt) . 2019 , 28(8):1031 -1036.

11. Choi K, Records K, Low L, Alhusen J, Kenner C, Bloch J et al. Promotion of Maternal–Infant Mental Health and Trauma-Informed Care During the COVID-19 Pandemic. Journal of Obstetric, Gynecologic & Neonatal Nursing. 2020;49(5):409-415.

www.ingramcontent.com/pod-product-compliance
Lightning Source LLC
Chambersburg PA
CBHW020917180526
45163CB00007B/2770